THE
INFLAMMATION
REVOLUTION

THE
INFLAMMATION
REVOLUTION

A Natural Solution for Arthritis, Asthma, & Other Inflammatory Disorders

Georges M. Halpern, MD, PhD

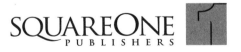

SQUAREONE
PUBLISHERS

The information and advice contained in this book are based upon the research and the personal and professional experiences of the author. They are not intended as a substitute for consulting with a health care professional. The publisher and author are not responsible for any adverse effects or consequences resulting from the use of any of the suggestions, preparations, or procedures discussed in this book. All matters pertaining to your physical health should be supervised by a health care professional. It is a sign of wisdom, not cowardice, to seek a second or third opinion.

Cover Designer: Jacqueline Michelus
Typesetter: Gary A. Rosenberg

Square One Publishers
115 Herricks Road
Garden City Park, NY 11040
(516) 535-2010 • (877) 900-BOOK
www.squareonepublishers.com

Library of Congress Cataloging-in-Publication Data

Halpern, Georges M.
   The inflammation revolution : a natural solution for arthritis, asthma, and other inflammatory disorders / Georges M. Halpern.
      p. cm.
   Includes bibliographical references and index.
   ISBN 0-7570-0283-8
   1. Arthritis—Alternative treatment. 2. Mussels. 3. Fish oils—Therapeutic use. 4. Anti-inflammatory agents. 5. Omega-3 fatty acids—Therapeutic use. I. Title.

RC933. H334 2005
616.7'2206—dc22

                                                                2005015966

Printed in the United States of America

10   9   8   7   6   5   4   3

Contents

Acknowledgments

I must first thank all the physicians, scientists, nurses, and patients whose lives, experiences, and research made this book possible. Many thanks also to Robert L. Meyer and John D. Waitzer, who have supported my work with the green-lipped mussel lipid oil extract. Krista Edmonds, PhD, was the superb researcher and outstanding writer who helped me with the first version of this book. Rudy Shur and his crew at Square One Publishers made this updated and revamped book available in record time (this contrasts with previous frustrating experiences in the profession). And finally, many, many thanks to my wife, Emiko, for her resilience, patience, and tolerance of the competing computer.

THE INFLAMMATION REVOLUTION

Introduction

"Oh, my aching knees . . ."
"You know, it's just aging. The old joints begin to hurt."
"It's my arthritis, dear. I can't knit or play the piano anymore."
"I don't remember the last time I went jogging. The arthritis is so bad."

D o any of these statements sound familiar? If so, you're typical of millions of Americans who suffer from an inflammatory condition, such as arthritis, or who have helplessly watched the suffering of arthritic parents or grandparents. Perhaps you have tried over-the-counter or even prescription medication to ease the pain. But if you're like many others, you've found that the benefits of these costly drugs are short-term at best. Worse, they are often fraught with unpleasant side effects. "Isn't there a better way?" you've wondered. The answer is "yes," and *The Inflammation Revolution* is designed to show you that better way. It's a way that brings together the ancient legends and practices of a small New Zealand tribe with the discoveries and technological advances of today's most sophisticated scientists and manufacturers. This book will introduce you to a health miracle from the sea—an oil derived from the green-lipped mussel that has been shown to have great anti-inflammatory benefits

Although inflammation has long been known as a cause of arthritis, recent scientific studies have uncovered its role in a number of other serious health conditions, including asthma, allergies,

1

and even heart attacks. Never before has there been such a need to understand the negative effects of inflammation. Just as critical is becoming aware of the dangers associated with its pharmaceutical remedies. Finally, and perhaps most important, is knowing the natural treatments available for managing inflammatory conditions—gently, safely, and effectively.

LEGENDARY CURE FROM THE SEA

The Maoris are an ancient tribe native to New Zealand. They have claimed for centuries that consuming green-lipped mussels raw helps them maintain good health. The reported incidence of arthritis is extremely low among the coastal-dwelling Maoris, who consume large amounts of raw green-lipped mussels, whereas Maoris who reside in the interior areas of the country have the same incidence of arthritis as New Zealanders of European origin. This combination of ancient legend and careful observation of the Maoris' actual health patterns intrigued researchers in the United Kingdom, Australia, Austria, and Japan. They decided to investigate the mussels' reported anti-inflammatory activity. Eventually, the efforts of these researchers yielded an oil extracted from the green-lipped mussel, and currently available in supplement form.

Since the early 1990s, clinical studies have shown that the oil from green-lipped mussels is a highly effective anti-inflammatory for relieving the symptoms of arthritis. These findings make sense in light of earlier research into the biochemistry of inflammation. Researchers have known that marine lipids (fats derived from fish) are actually the best and most available source of fat in some areas of the world. They have also known that these marine lipids, regardless of their structure, have some protective, anti-inflammatory effects on blood vessels and joints, and may also provide benefits to other organs, such as the skin, lungs, and gastrointestinal tract.

The traditions of people around the world confirm this scientific knowledge: people who eat fatty fish enjoy better health. The benefits of fish oil were known not only in primitive cultures, but in Western societies as well. Your great-grandparents, for example, may have swallowed a spoonful of cod-liver oil before school or before bedtime. As a child, hiding in Savoie, France, during World War II, I also took cod-liver oil regularly—and loved it! I wasn't sure why it was beneficial; I just knew it was "good for me" and that it also tasted wonderful.

What's so special about the green-lipped mussel? As the saying goes, we are what we eat. This is true for all living organisms, not just for human beings. Even the tiny creatures that produce marine lipids are influenced by what *they* eat. Their diet consists of one-celled organisms called plankton. The particular population of plankton that the green-lipped mussels feed on is exposed to higher than normal levels of radiation. As a result, the plankton has adapted by producing high levels of antioxidants as a means of protection. When the green-lipped mussels ingest this plankton, they absorb the same protection. So, while all fish oils are beneficial, the lipid extract in these particular mussels is higher in antioxidants than most others. Additionally, the New Zealand government zealously protects the waters in which these mussels live, keeping them free of contaminants that affect fish from other regions of the world.

You don't necessarily have to use the oil extract to reap health benefits. You can also eat these delicious mussels raw as part of your daily diet. They are considered delicacies and are sold all over the world. In fact, they are a staple in the best restaurants and fish markets around the globe. Traditionally, the Maori people eat them raw. Although you can certainly cook them if you prefer, they will lose their nutraceutical benefits in the process. If you do not enjoy eating seafood products, have difficulty obtaining green-lipped mussels locally, or want more exact guidelines regarding quantities and dosages, you can take the lipid oil extract. This supplement yields the same health benefits as the raw mussels.

A VARIETY OF HEALTH BENEFITS

Researchers have found that the green-lipped mussel oil extract, which contains healthy omega-3 polyunsaturated fatty acids, is one of the best anti-inflammatory agents available. Most chronic diseases that afflict people in industrialized western societies have an inflammatory component. Treatment options are not always ideal, and this lipid extract may be beneficial to many people who suffer from these diseases.

Arthritis, for example, costs Americans some $65 billion per year in treatment costs and lost productivity. Current research shows that both osteoarthritis and rheumatoid arthritis respond to the mussel oil extract with significant reductions in inflammation and swelling. Moreover, this mussel oil extract has been found to be nontoxic and free of significant side effects. Unlike most medications used to treat arthritis—such as non-steroidal anti-inflammatory drugs (NSAIDs), which have adverse gastrointestinal side effects—the oil extract of green-lipped mussels actually *protects* the gastrointestinal tract.

In addition to its positive anti-inflammatory effects, this lipid oil is also helpful in the prevention of cardiovascular problems. While this is true of most fish oils, this mussel oil is considered safer for those with circulatory problems. This is because other fish oils, which inhibit blood clotting, may result in excessive bleeding in case of injury. The oil from green-lipped mussels, however, does not affect clotting. This means it is completely safe for menstruating women, as well as for anyone already taking blood thinners, such as aspirin.

This lipid oil extract also shows promise as an anti-asthma and anti-allergy treatment. Asthma affects an estimated 17 million Americans, including nearly 5 million children. It is responsible for nearly half a million hospitalizations, over 1 million emergency room visits, and more than 5,000 deaths annually, at a cost of approximately $6.2 billion per year. Studies from around the world have shown that green-lipped mussel oil reduces asthma symptoms due to its anti-inflammatory effects on airways leading to the lungs. It has been found safer than today's pharmaceuticals for asthma, including the newer medications that are supposed to be relatively free of side effects.

Even the skin can benefit from this lipid oil extract, which protects against radiation and also slows the skin's natural aging process. The carotenoids and omega-3 fatty acids present in this extract are essential for healthy skin. Like other fish oils, which contain essential fatty acids associated with skin protection, this lipid oil extract speeds wound healing and prevents excessive scarring.

While the list of health benefits provided by green-lipped mussel oil is already impressive, ongoing research continues to expand our understanding of this extract and its positive applications for good health.

WHY *THE INFLAMMATION REVOLUTION?*

If you are suffering from any inflammatory disorder, *The Inflammation Revolution* will show you how the green-lipped mussel oil extract can help you. After an opening chapter that offers a brief glimpse into the history and characteristics of this lipid oil, the book reviews relevant research on it, as well as important issues surrounding the development of stabilized mussel preparations. Chapter 3 looks at inflammatory joint disease and arthritis, and shows how this oil extract can be effective in reducing symptoms of rheumatoid arthritis, as well as osteoarthritis. Chapter 4 focuses on the extract's positive effects on the cardiovascular system, while Chapter 5 discusses its effectiveness in treating asthma, allergies, and skin disorders. Chapter 6 takes a look at green-lipped mussel oil extract and the needs of women, specifically addressing how it can be helpful in alleviating menstrual discomforts. Chapter 7 offers a tantalizing glimpse into the future by reviewing the current research on new applications of this extraordinary oil. Concluding the book, Chapter 8 provides usage guidelines for the extract.

With the risks of many anti-inflammatory prescription drugs continuing to make headlines, it has become vital for the millions who suffer from arthritis and other inflammatory conditions to find safer options. Backed by scientific evidence, *The Inflammation Revolution* shows how the oil extract from green-lipped mussels works and—most important—how this "miracle from the sea" can be used to safely and effectively relieve the pain and suffering of inflammatory conditions.

1

The Secret of the Green-Lipped Mussel

A bout 1,000 years ago, the Maoris arrived in New Zealand. It appears that they began to consume large quantities of green-lipped mussels during the fifteenth century, when an extended cold period forced them to spend whole summers fishing along the coast and smoke-drying their catch for storage. When the climate warmed up again (approximately during the sixteenth century), heavy rainfall and gale-force winds increased flooding and made life on the coast uncomfortable. It appears that as they moved farther inland, they retained their taste for seafood.

Their strong attachment to the green-lipped mussel, however, was not merely a matter of taste. They believed, as modern-day Maoris continue to believe, that consuming these mussels helped them maintain good health. Today, we know that their belief was no mere superstition—there are scientifically proven reasons for their good health.

Europeans started to arrive in New Zealand in the mid-1600s, beginning with the Dutch explorer Abel Tasman and English mariner Captain James Cook. After this, the flow of Europeans never stopped. When European settlers began to arrive in New Zealand in significant numbers during the nineteenth century, they brought with them their European diseases as well as their bad health habits, including the European diet and the use of alcohol and tobacco.

The Maori population fell from about 120,000 in 1769 to 42,000 in 1896. A major factor in their dwindling numbers was poor resistance to diseases such as smallpox, influenza, German measles, tuberculosis, whooping cough, typhoid, and sexually transmitted diseases. Medical assistance was scarce. Even when sparse medical resources could be marshaled, they usually reached the rural Maoris too late to save lives. Maoris also succumbed to alcohol abuse and experienced all its resultant problems. The introduction of the musket added a new devastation to the Maoris' own land battles. By the late nineteenth century, the European settlers were referring to the Maoris as "a dying race."

While most Maoris soon fell prey to European ailments, coastal Maoris appeared to be healthier. In particular, they did not suffer from arthritis as their European counterparts did. Anecdotal evidence and folk wisdom attribute this health benefit to the heavy consumption of raw green-lipped mussels.

MEET *PERNA CANALICULUS*

No, this is not a Latin lesson. You're being formally introduced to the green-lipped mussel, using its correct biological name, *Perna canaliculus*, which—like all scientific names of living creatures—is Latin. There is a new patented, stabilized natural marine lipid oil from the New Zealand green-lipped mussel. It contains a rare combination of lipid (fat) groups containing both known and unknown polyunsaturated fatty acids (PUFAs). You'll learn more about these ingredients later, but for now, let's just say that the known PUFAs, which include omega-3s and some eicosatetraenoic acids (ETAs), have been shown to be extremely powerful anti-inflammatory compounds that are particularly effective against arthritis.

Why is this lipid oil so effective? It is a purer product than most fish oils because the green-lipped mussel lives in such a sheltered and protected environment. The lipids found in the green-lipped mussel are especially rich and efficacious due to a combination of the mussels' genetics and their food—tiny organisms called microplankton. The plankton that the mussels feed on are rich in antioxidants because of the amount of sunlight that falls upon the waters where they live. The sun's rays are unusually intense and, in order to survive, the plankton must protect themselves from the high levels of ultraviolet (UV) radiation, which can reach potentially deadly levels. They have evolved to fight oxidative stress caused by radiation with powerful antioxidants. The mussels, in turn, absorb these protective mechanisms when they ingest the plankton. When you eat the raw mussels—or their extracted oil— you absorb the wonderful protective properties of the plankton.

FROM MAORI SECRET TO WESTERN SCIENCE

Interest in the green-lipped mussel began when it was noticed that the coastal Maoris had far less arthritis than the inland Maoris. A company from Australia began investigating the health benefits of the New Zealand green-lipped mussel in the 1970s and spearheaded the pioneering work that eventually led to the production of this specific lipid oil.

The first products produced from the New Zealand green-lipped mussel were various preparations of dried mussel powder. These preparations were less than ideal because they were unstable and oxidized rapidly, they held residual moisture, and they had a characteristic odor that many people found offensive.

By 1975, a new freeze-dried powder extract became available. It was less malodorous and therefore became considerably more popular. However, hard scientific evidence supporting the extract was still lacking. By 1978, manufacturers of the mussel powder extract were actively seeking scientific validation that the extract could be helpful in reducing symptoms of arthritis. They succeeded in piquing the interest of Drs. Robin Gibson and Sheila Gibson, a Scottish husband-and-wife medical team, who conducted the first major study. Their results, published in *The Practitioner* in 1980, showed clearly that the mussel powder extract had a substantial effect on certain forms of arthritis.

Unfortunately, the Gibsons' results, though promising, were not easily replicated. The discrepancy between study findings turned out to be caused by the fact that the clinical studies utilized unstable, rather than the stabilized, mussel powder. The stabilized powder could protect against oxidation, but the unstabilized could not. European manufacturers, who sell unstabilized powder, use the same brand name—Seatone—as the Australian and Japanese manufacturers who use stabilized powder. The unstablized product has given the lipid extract a bad reputation. Until 1983, researchers studying the effects of the mussel powder extract experienced considerable variations in the level of anti-inflammatory activity from batch to batch due to poor stability. Today, the stabilized powder is readily available and is the superior product.

The Australian company, convinced that the mussels contained some potent active ingredient, began research to identify what that ingredient might be and to isolate it. In 1992, Dr. W. Henry Betts, the principal scientist at the Rheumatology Research Laboratory of the Queen Elizabeth Hospital, in Adelaide, South Australia, discovered some very active compounds in mussel extract. Dr. Betts, who used an *in vitro* method of testing anti-inflammatory compounds, was amazed to discover that some of the substances in the green-lipped mussel powder were the most potent in his laboratory. Unfortunately, they were not pure enough for him to identify.

His interest had been captured, however, and he was not willing to let the implications of these findings slip away from him. His enthusiasm led him to introduce the Australian entrepreneurs of the New Zealand mussel to Dr. Michael W. Whitehouse, an expert in testing for anti-inflammatory activity in laboratory animals. In 1994, Dr. Whitehouse's animal studies confirmed the activity of the stabilized green-lipped mussel powder extract.

PRODUCING THE GREEN-LIPPED MUSSEL LIPID OIL

Having identified active ingredients, the next obstacle was finding a way to extract the compounds commercially without damaging them. It took two more years of intensive testing to develop the patented process. The mussels are harvested from the pristine waters of the Marlborough Sound of New Zealand by specifically equipped ships, which are totally enclosed so they release no pollution. In less than two hours, the mussels—which are kept under maximum refrigeration to ensure freshness—reach the grinder and centrifuge at the factory. They go through a series of processes to extract their essential liquid, which is combined with a stabilizing natural fruit acid and freeze-dried. This freeze-dried stabilized powder of mussel is produced using Good Manufacturing Practices as defined by the food industry and approved by the United States Food and Drug Administration (FDA). The stabilized mussel powder is then shipped to a laboratory, where the oil is extracted through a liquid carbon dioxide process instead of chemical solvents. It is then combined with pharmaceutical-grade olive oil (50 mg of lipid extract and 100 mg of olive oil) and encapsulated. The end product is the lipid oil extract of green-lipped mussels— a concentrated and stabilized dietary supplement.

Once processed from stabilized mussel powder, the lipid oil extract is easily digestible; it does not contain any salt, so patients with high blood pressure or anyone adhering to a low-sodium diet can safely use it. Lipid oil extract has no protein; it also has no carbohydrates, making it safe for diabetics. It contains unique fatty acids that help reduce inflammation in the body. Other anti-inflammatory agents identified in the lipid oil extract of green-lipped mussels are carotenoids. Carotenoids circulate through the body, scavenging for free radicals and protecting against oxidative damage.

2

Dietary Fats and the Green-Lipped Mussel Lipid Oil

Can diet influence disease? The idea of a connection between what we eat and how healthy we are has been explored throughout history in numerous cultures, both primitive and modern. Obviously, ancient peoples understood that eating certain foods—say, poisonous mushrooms—led to acute illnesses or death. But even among the ancients, myths and legends abounded regarding the impact of diet on health. In today's world, the connection between diet and chronic illnesses such as heart disease and diabetes is obvious and wholly accepted in popular and scientific circles.

Only in the last two or three decades, however, have scientists become aware of the connection between diet and other diseases. Researchers are linking diet to cancer as well as to inflammatory diseases. They are discovering that lifestyle and diet are even more important than family history in determining who succumbs to many chronic diseases. Studies of immigrants show that the rate of disease among populations changes as their environment changes—their new lifestyles are probably as important as their genetic profile.

A good example of this is the incidence of heart disease and breast cancer among the Japanese. Japanese people living in their own country and adhering to their traditional diet—which is low in animal fats and high in brown rice and vegetable proteins such as tofu—have relatively few cases of heart disease and breast cancer. Japanese people living in Hawaii, who have included more "American" foods in their diet, have a higher incidence of these diseases, while Japanese living on the West Coast of the United States have the highest incidence of all. This disturbing trend is clearly related to the Americanization of their diet.

While America is one of the wealthiest countries in the world, affluence has not translated itself into better health. Quite the contrary: a sedentary lifestyle, combined with the easy availability of foods high in animal fat, sugars, and chemicals, has led to an array of diseases. Cardiovascular disease, cancer, and arthritis top the list. However, other conditions are rising significantly, including rheumatoid arthritis, multiple sclerosis, chronic fatigue syndrome, inflammatory bowel disorders (such as ulcerative colitis and Crohn's disease), diabetes, fibromyalgia, lupus erythematosus, some thyroid disorders, and scleroderma. These are called autoimmune disorders and arise when your immune system starts attacking structures within your own body.

Western science has fought back with an impressive array of drugs designed to suppress the immune system. While they are effective in controlling serious flare-ups of symptoms, they also cause almost as many problems as they solve. Suppressing your immune system means that you're more vulnerable to invasions of viruses and bacteria. The drugs can also damage healthy organs. And ultimately, they don't solve the problem. They merely relieve the symptoms for a little while—and only for as long as you take them.

Solid scientific research has begun to point us in the direction of lifestyle changes that *can* solve the problem or at least contribute to its solution. Reducing consumption of animal fats and increasing dietary intake of vegetables, fruits, and whole grains can decrease the inflammation that occurs in many autoimmune disorders. Eating deep-water fish instead of hamburgers, hydrogenated oils, and high-fat cheeses may make your joints less achy.

ALL DIETARY FATS ARE NOT CREATED EQUAL

All oils are not created equal, and all fat isn't bad. You may be surprised to learn that some fats are necessary for good health. Scientists have found that supplementing the diet with oils high in certain essential fatty acids (EFAs, such as omega-3 and some omega-6) is highly beneficial. Some of these "good" oils are plant-based, including flaxseed, rapeseed, borage, evening primrose, and canola oils. Small amounts of these "good" oils are also present in baked beans and most green leafy vegetables. Other healthful oils are fish based: cod-liver oil is perhaps the best-known example, but there are others as well.

Even among these beneficial oils, some are superior to others. When scientists compared the effects of dietary fish oil to dietary flaxseed oil, they found that the marine and vegetable oils were very similar in their beneficial effects. However, they also discovered that the omega-3 polyunsaturated fatty acids (PUFAs) contained in fish were five to ten times more efficacious than those found in plants. This means that very large amounts of flaxseed oil were needed to accomplish what relatively small quantities of fish oil managed to do—namely, to reduce elevated triacylglycerol levels in the blood. Triacylglycerols are lipids found in the blood—excessively high levels place a person at risk for diabetes and cardiovascular disease.

DISCOVERING THE BENEFITS OF FISH OILS

The growing body of evidence on the beneficial effects of omega-3 fatty acids makes it increasingly clear that fish is a much more important food than had previously been supposed. But scientists didn't come to this conclusion by jumping directly to a study of fish. They began by looking at PUFAs in general. American researchers identified two major categories of PUFAs as far back as the 1930s, omega-6 and omega-3 acids. It was discovered that linoleic acid is the parent or precursor for the omega-6 PUFAs, while alpha-linolenic acid is the parent fatty acid for the omega-3 PUFAs.

In 1972, two Danish scientists noticed that the Inuits of Greenland had a much lower incidence of death from coronary heart disease and other diseases associated with affluence than the other citizens of Greenland, despite a diet consisting mainly of seal fat. The blood fat levels of the Inuits were relatively low—a surprising finding considering their high-fat diet. In fact, their entire blood profile reflected a picture of good health, especially compared with Danes from Greenland whose diet was "Western." The researchers were baffled because these findings flew in the face of established beliefs about cholesterol levels and their effects on coronary heart disease. How could anyone live on seal fat and have such ideal cholesterol and triglyceride levels? Why weren't the Inuits suffering from heart attacks?

After much research, the two scientists concluded that the low incidence of heart disease could be attributed to the Inuits' marine diet. The unusual blood lipid profile of Greenland Inuits was consistent with reductions in heart attacks. They began to draw connections to other cultures and countries. For example, they noted that the incidence of heart disease and resulting death fell dramatically in Norway following the German invasion in 1940, when Norwegians shifted to a fish-based rather than a meat-based diet. Since this pioneering research, other scientists have studied dozens of cultures throughout the world and their findings confirm the association between a high-fish diet and a low incidence of cardiovascular disease.

A CLOSER LOOK AT DIETARY FATS

Let's take a closer look at omega-6 and omega-3 PUFAs in order to understand why the fats that dominate our Western diet tend to be so destructive, while fish-based fats are so healing. At the beginning of the twenty-first century, the type of dietary fat required for optimum health has become a confusing subject not only for consumers but for scientists as well. It is a controversial subject, and it seems that every few months there's a new report of some scientific finding concerning fat that appears to contradict the last finding.

Although fats and oils have been part of the human diet since the beginning of recorded time, scientific study of dietary fats has lagged behind the study of proteins and carbohydrates during the development of nutritional science. In fact, fat was not even recognized as an important nutrient until 1827. Only in the 1900s was fat recognized as a source of abundant energy as well as a vehicle for the metabolism of fat-soluble vitamins. The concept of "essential fatty acids" is a relatively recent phenomenon.

As Western consumption of animal fat (mainly lard and butter) increased dramatically through the beginning of the twentieth century, the study of fat became more urgent. Epidemiologists correlated high levels of blood cholesterol, linked to the high consumption of animal fats, with the prevalence of coronary heart disease. Eventually, people began altering their diet, reducing consumption of animal fats and switching to other fats that supposedly were less destructive.

Margarine was touted as a healthful alternative to butter, for example. People began to believe that if they avoided egg yolks and red meat, nibbling instead on margarine sandwiches, they would have a healthy blood profile. The main PUFA in the Western food supply became linoleic acid, the precursor of the omega-6 series, and the major fatty acid found in most vegetable oils and margarine. This "solution" generated unforeseen consequences, however, leading to an entirely new set of health problems.

The main problem was that people were now consuming large quantities of omega-6 fatty acids. This fatty acid is not in and of itself destructive and, in fact, it is very effective at lowering blood cholesterol levels. What is destructive, however, is eating so much of it and eating so little of the omega-3 fatty acids. These are equally essential but are not present at very high levels in most Western diets.

Large quantities of omega-6 fatty acids created a new imbalance in dietary fats. The high level of omega-6 relative to omega-3 PUFAs in the Western diet (a ratio of about 15:1 or higher) is due to a diet enriched in linoleic acid from sources such as margarine and salad oils. Prior to the widespread use of omega-6 vegetable oils in the food supply, the omega-6/omega-3 ratio in diets was closer to 1:1. Consumption of these oils has risen dramatically— and, ironically, because people believe that these fats are good for their health. This, however, isn't true and the glut of omega-6 vegetable oils has caused a sharp rise in cardiovascular disease.

A BALANCING ACT

The balance between the omega-6 and omega-3 essential fatty acids has become increasingly central to our understanding of good health. Both groups serve as precursors for a host of chemicals that perform necessary functions in the body. Some of the chemicals that are derived from the omega-6 and omega-3 groups are prostaglandins, prostacyclins, thromboxanes, and leukotrienes. All these complicated-sounding substances are crucial to our good health—they affect our immune systems, circulatory systems, and joints. When they are correctly balanced, we remain healthy. Our joints do not become inflamed and arthritic. The membranes in our airways also remain free of inflammation, so we do not suffer from asthma. The mucosal lining in our digestive tract is protected, so we avoid irritable bowel syndrome or other inflammatory digestive disorders. Our blood fat (cholesterol and triglyceride) levels are healthy, preventing heart attacks, strokes, and other cardiovascular problems. And our circulation remains normal, so we don't suffer from thrombosis.

The omega-6 group contains large quantities of linoleic acid (LA), a precursor chemical for arachidonic acid, which, in turn, leads to the production of many other chemicals. When these chemicals are overproduced, they can have numerous negative effects. The omega-3 group, on the other hand, is rich in alpha-linolenic acid (ALA), which is a precursor to two other EFAs—eicosapentaenoic acid (EPA) and docosahexaenoic acid (DHA). These have the opposite effect of arachidonic acid; they inhibit production of the substances that arachidonic acid generally stimulates. This system of checks and balances works quite well. Arachidonic acid causes the production of important substances, while EPA and DHA make sure that these substances are not overproduced.

For example, scientists studying thrombosis—a condition that occurs when a blood clot is lodged within a blood vessel—discovered that the key to maintaining healthy blood vessels lies in maintaining a balance between two chemicals in the body. One is called thromboxane 2 (TXA_2), which causes blood cells to clump together and blood vessels to tighten and constrict. We need this substance so that when we cut ourselves, our blood will clot and a scab will form. Constricted blood vessels reduce the amount of blood that reaches the area, thereby minimizing blood loss.

On the other hand, we don't want blood clots moving through our arteries and veins. They block the flow of blood, causing numerous problems at the site of the clot. Even worse, they travel and a blood clot that reaches the heart can be fatal. So the body balances out TXA_2 by producing another chemical called prostacyclin (PGI_2). This works against the clotting of blood and also promotes dilation, or widening, of the blood vessels.

For us to remain healthy, a correct balance of both these chemicals must be maintained. Thrombosis occurs when the balance is disrupted and TXA_2 is not counterbalanced by sufficient quantities of PGI_2. One of the discoveries about the Greenland Inuits was that their blood was rich in EPA, which helps maintain the balance between TXA_2 and PGI_2. The Danes, on the other hand, had hardly any detectable levels of EPA in their blood at all. Researchers have since established that increased consumption of fish oil leads to increased production of PGI_2, resulting in the remarkable lack of thrombosis and other circulatory difficulties among the Eskimos.

As mentioned above, marine-based omega-3 oils have been shown to be superior to plant-based oils. Their benefits are associated not only with preventing cardiovascular disease but also with reduction in inflammatory disorders, such as arthritis. For example, arachidonic acid leads to the production of leukotrienes. These are beneficial substances and they accomplish a host of necessary functions in the body. Believe it or not, inflammation is an example of a necessary function—it is your body's way of fighting unwelcome and potentially dangerous invading organisms. Too many leukotrienes, however, lead to unnecessary and counterproductive inflammation. Inflammatory disorders such as arthritis, asthma, and irritable bowel syndrome are all associated with excessive production of leukotrienes. Omega-3 PUFAs control leukotriene production, leading to a reduction in inflammation. All the omega-3 PUFAs are helpful in inhibiting leukotrienes, but fish oil is more efficacious than plant-based oil, and the green-lipped mussel oil extract is the most powerful anti-inflammatory marine oil available.

UNIQUE FATS IN GREEN-LIPPED MUSSELS

Fish oil is highly beneficial, but all fish oils are not equally beneficial. The marine food chain is dominated by omega-3 PUFAs: fish, shellfish, and other fish products such as fish eggs (roe) or oils (cod-liver oil) are the main sources of marine-based omega-3s in our diet. Research has shown that the lipid oil extract of green-lipped mussels is superior to oils derived from fish and roe and even to oils derived from other shellfish.

The secret lies in its unique ingredients. The oil from the green-lipped mussel has properties not found in any other marine sources. In fact, it is 200 times more effective at reducing the swelling of arthritis in laboratory animals than other fish oils that contain more run-of-the-mill PUFAs. The active ingredients of the lipid oil extract of green-lipped mussels are a series of unique omega-3 PUFAs called eicosatetraenoic acids (ETAs). A critical review conducted at two universities in Australia found that these ingredients are responsible for its effectiveness. The lipid oil extract of green-lipped mussels stands alone in its ability to successfully control leukotrienes, which are responsible for initiating and spreading inflammation throughout the body.

Inflammation is one of the ways in which the body controls infection and promotes healing. In the right context, the body's ability to produce inflammation is actually critical to good health, but you can also have too much of a good thing and it becomes a problem. In the case of arthritis, asthma, and similar conditions, the process goes awry and the body fights itself: it sends out its inflammatory "soldiers" to fight interior "friends" instead of invading external "enemies." Conditions such as rheumatoid arthritis and asthma are therefore called autoimmune diseases, in which the body is producing "immunity" against itself.

Leukotrienes (a group of the chemicals that cause inflammation) are released by healthy individuals to combat illness, but those who suffer from autoimmune diseases produce too many leukotrienes. There are two major pathways responsible for inflammation in the body: These are the LOX (lipoxygenase) pathway and the COX (cyclo-oxygenase) pathway. Both pathways function by producing a chemical called arachidonate, which is responsible for oxygenization (the addition of oxygen to form a new substance). The new substances formed by the LOX pathway are the leukotrienes. The COX pathway produces other inflammatory substances called prostaglandins and thromboxanes. When either or both of these pathways malfunction, producing excessive leukotrienes, prostaglandins, or thromboxanes, inflammation results. You wake up groaning with arthritic pain or wheezing with asthma, for example.

Current anti-inflammatory medications, the non-steroidal anti-inflammatory drugs or NSAIDs (for a current list, see Appendix A, beginning on page 111), function by inhibiting the COX pathway. As mentioned, these drugs can have serious side effects. What's more, they don't address inflammatory activity caused by the LOX pathway. So, scientists are turning their attention to developing inhibitors of the LOX pathway. A new class of drugs called anti-leukotrienes is being used to address asthma, but these do not address COX activity. This means that many asthmatics have to take several medications, with an array of side effects.

Is there a substance that can inhibit *both* the LOX and the COX pathways? The answer is yes—the lipid oil of green-lipped mussels inhibits both these inflammatory pathways. The lipid oil's wide range of impressive results may be attributed to the fact that it is actually not a single substance. There are a variety of active ingredients contained in green-lipped mussels, over and above the fatty acids that have so far been identified. For example, there are about ten different marine sterols (a kind of oil) and more than thirty fatty acids—saturated, monounsaturated, and polyunsaturated—in the lipid extract. Each of these ingredients has a different effect on the COX or LOX pathways.

Unsaturated fatty acids present in the lipid oil of green-lipped mussels have emerged as new, previously unidentified substances that work against the metabolism of arachidonate. They work synergistically with other oils, such as EPA and DHA, that are present in many marine foods. The result is a powerful combination of substances that inhibits metabolism of arachidonates produced by *both* pathways. Perhaps this is the reason why smaller quantities of the lipid extract are required to bring about anti-inflammatory results. There are more fatty acids present and they strengthen and enhance one another's effectiveness.

One particular omega-3 fatty acid in the green-lipped mussel, called omega-3 tetraenoic, is virtually identical to arachidonic acid, which is the agent responsible for acting on the COX and LOX pathways to produce inflammation. This fatty acid can "fool" the pathways into "believing" that they are bonding with arachidonic acid, with the result that inflammatory agents, such as leuko-trienes, are not produced.

Plus, the lipid oil of the green-lipped mussel is free of side effects. It appears that the fatty acids in the lipid oil can distinguish between different aspects of the COX pathway and target only those responsible for inflammation. The COX pathway actually consists of two components, COX-1 and COX-2. COX-1 is a "house-keeper" responsible for upkeep of the areas in the body that have protective mucous linings, including the digestive tract. COX-2 is responsible for inflammation. Unlike NSAIDs, the lipid oil of green-lipped mussels suppresses COX-2 while leaving COX-1 untouched. So, there are no unpleasant digestive side effects.

In fact, you can't really overdose on the lipid oil. Researchers in Australia tried to induce some kind of negative reaction in mice by giving them megadoses of lipid oil but didn't manage to kill even a single mouse. So it works, and it's safe.

A REVIEW OF SCIENTIFIC STUDIES

Many scientific studies have focused on the lipid oil extract of green-lipped mussels and most unequivocally support its effec-tiveness. Many studies also point to the superiority of the green-lipped mussel oil over conventional medications, plant-based omega-3 oils, and even over other marine oils. These studies will be discussed in greater detail in the chapters on each disease con-dition, but we'll look at a few of the studies here.

- A randomized study conducted at Glasgow Hospital in Scotland found that green-lipped mussel lipid oil inhibited leukotriene synthesis, reducing the severity of a particular form of arthritis in laboratory rats.

- Studies conducted at Queen Elizabeth Hospital in Adelaide, Australia, demonstrated that the oil extract inhibits activity of the LOX pathway, reducing the damaging effects of persistent inflammation and bringing relief to those who suffer from allergic reactions, including asthma. The studies also supported the effectiveness of green-lipped mussel oil extract in bringing about relief from arthritis symptoms.

- A study conducted at the University of Queensland in Australia tested the anti-arthritis properties of the green-lipped mussel lipid oil extract by measuring various arthritis symptoms in laboratory rats. The lipid oil reduced joint swelling by 91%, compared to untreated rats, which experienced no reduction in swelling. It was 200 to 350 times as effective as other oils used to treat inflammation—at one-hundredth the dosage. The scientists compared the lipid oil with indomethacin and ibuprofen, two widely used anti-arthritis drugs. At the same dose rate, the lipid oil outperformed both by a factor of two to one.

- A randomized clinical trial of green-lipped mussel oil extract was conducted in Scotland involving 30 participants with classic rheumatoid arthritis and 30 with clinical evidence of osteoarthritis. Both groups showed significant improvement with the lipid oil.

- A pilot study conducted in Denmark on patients suffering from osteoarthritis showed that lipid oil dramatically decreased the level of pain in a two- to three-month period.

- A study, conducted at the Queen Mary Hospital of the University of Hong Kong, compared the effects of the green-lipped mussel oil extract versus placebo on the signs and symptoms and quality of life in patients with osteoarthritis (OA) of the knee. Eighty patients with knee OA were randomized to receive either the mussel extract or placebo for six months. Improvement in almost all of the arthritis assessment variables was observed in both groups of patients. However, there was a significantly greater improvement in the perception of pain (VAS) and patient's global assessment of OA in those who took the mussel oil extract.

- Researchers in Seoul, South Korea, organized a multi-center two-month clinical trial with a total of eight specialized clinics. Sixty patients with symptomatic, painful OA of the knee and hip received mussel oil extract at a dose of two capsules twice daily. After a four- and eight-week treatment period, 53% and 80% of patients experienced significant pain relief and improvement of joint function, respectively. There were no reported adverse effects attributable to the oil extract.

- Recently, Dr. Michael W. Whitehouse of the University of Queensland, Australia, suggested the symbiotic association of pentoxiphylline, an inhibitor of the pro-inflammatory cytokine TNF-alpha, with mussel oil extract as an effective treatment of active inflammatory arthritis and a prednisone/corticosteroid–sparing strategy.

- In Germany, a group of physicians studied the efficacy and tolerability of a combination of the lipid oil extract of green-lipped mussels and high concentrations of EPA and DHA in patients with rheumatoid arthritis (RA). This twelve-week drug-monitoring study was conducted on 50 adults, men and women. A total of 34 patients required important drug therapy before and during the study. But by the end of the study, 21 (62%) were able to reduce their dosage and, more importantly, 13 were able to terminate all medications. At week twelve, 38% were symptom free, and the number of patients complaining of severe pain decreased significantly from 60% to 25% at the completion of the trial.

- Asthma is a chronic inflammatory disease of the airways mediated, at least in part, by leukotrienes and other lipid mediators. A study at the Pavlov Medical University in St. Petersburg, Russia, assessed the effects of green-lipped mussel oil extract on the symptoms of asthma. Forty-six patients with atopic asthma received two capsules of the lipid oil or a placebo twice daily for eight weeks. At the end of the study, there was a significant decrease in daytime wheeze, in the concentration of exhaled hydrogen peroxide, and an increase in morning peak expiratory flow.

- Researchers in St. Petersburg, Russia, and Melbourne, Australia, studied the effects of the lipid extract in patients receiving a nasal spray of live, attenuated influenza vaccine. The mussel oil extract possessed significant immunomodulating effects on post-vaccination immune responses in those vaccinated with live influenza vaccine. It proved to be a safe stimulant in these subjects.

- Dietary supplementation with the lipid oil induced, after six weeks, a significant increase in the content of omega-3 fatty acids in neutrophils, together with a significant reduction of inflammation-associated mediators, according to researchers at the RMIT University in Melbourne, Australia. This study implied that the lipid oil should be part of a prevention program for aging and chronic inflammatory disease, including cardiovascular disease.

- Other studies compared the lipid oil extract of green-lipped mussels to other oils—flaxseed oil, evening primrose oil, salmon oil, and Max-EPA (a combination fish-oil product)—claiming to have anti-arthritic properties. The researchers used an equal dosage of each oil and measured the effect of each agent in controlling joint swelling associated with arthritis. As you can see from the following results, the lipid oil extract of green-lipped mussels proved to be the most effective. It was:
  - 200 times more potent than Max-EPA.
  - 250 times more potent than unprocessed green-lipped mussel extract.
  - 350 times more potent than evening primrose oil.
  - 350 times more potent than salmon oil.
  - 400 times more potent than flaxseed oil.

The combined findings of all of these studies point to the lipid oil extract of green-lipped mussels as the most effective agent in reducing arthritis symptoms and inflammation. It is superior to conventional pharmaceuticals, vegetable-based omega-3 oils, other fish oils, and even the unprocessed extract of the green-lipped mussel.

BALANCING YOUR FAT INTAKE

There are two different approaches to oils: one focuses on the amount of oils consumed and the other looks at the types of oils consumed. Certainly it is valuable to examine how much oil you're actually consuming on a regular basis. Do you cook with oil? Do you incorporate it into cakes and breads? Do you use spreads, such as butter or margarine, which are fatty? Is fat a favorite ingredient of your salad dressing? You can tally up how much oil you ingest by estimating how many tablespoons you eat every day from all these varied sources. Many studies have shown that a high-fat diet contributes to cancer, cardiovascular disease, and a host of other dangerous conditions.

However, don't go to the other extreme and completely shun all fat. Remember that you need essential fatty acids, which are not produced by your own body. You need both omega-6 and omega-3 fatty acids, but you don't need to pour enormous quantities of oil into your mouth—or your frying pan. Remember that fatty acids work like medicine in your system. When you take a drug, you don't take huge quantities—you usually can swallow a small pill, containing just the right quantity of active ingredients. These powerful substances shoot through your body like missiles, going right to your body's receptors to do their job, creating appropriate reactions in your body.

You know that many medications can have serious and even life-threatening consequences when taken in excess. Fats should be regarded as "medications" that can be unhealthful when taken in excess. While the part you need is absorbed and used by the body, the excess is not excreted but stored. Some is stored in your body's cells and is the part that contributes to unsightly weight problems. Some is stored along and within blood vessels, contributing to atherosclerosis.

You don't want to eat too much fat, nor do you want to completely eliminate fat. The key is to eat healthful fats in appropriate quantities and in correct balance.

Let's look at the physiology of most natural fats. If you shine a light through a slide of fat in liquid form or in a very thin solid form, the light will be diverted. If the light moves toward you, it's called a *cis-fatty* acid. However, if you hydrogenate or heat your oils, the light moves away from you and you get a *trans-fatty* acid. The trans-fatty acids (or hydrogenated oils) have been shown to be irritants. In fact, they are pro-inflammatory *if* they are consumed by themselves. Margarine and most shortenings are trans-fatty acids. Baked goods contain lots of trans-fatty acids because they become solid at room temperature and resist heat very well, thereby extending the shelf life of products. When they are absorbed and metabolized in the body, they give rise to more arachidonic acid precursors, which are the precursors of inflammatory substances. Trans-fatty acids also damage the inner layer of your small arteries, creating inflammation of the artery that will eventually lead to cardiovascular disease.

It's hard to get away from these fats. They seem to be present in just about everything, especially our favorite foods. However, it is crucial to cut down on them because of their destructive effects. This does not mean that we have to completely eliminate them. Try to use unprocessed, expeller-pressed oils—especially monounsaturated oils, such as olive and canola. These work nicely alone and even better in combination. Canola oil can be heated at a higher temperature than olive oil without becoming bitter and potentially toxic.

Just as important, using these oils will help counterbalance your intake of omega-6 fatty acids by increasing your intake of omega-3 fatty acids. This will offset some of the negative results of the trans-fatty acids. They will also provide the balance we discussed earlier between the omega-6 and omega-3 acids, so that they function most optimally in your body.

Some research has suggested that there is metabolic competition between omega-3 and omega-6 PUFAs, as if each is trying to "elbow" the other aside and claim its place in the sun. The implication is that omega-6 PUFAs derived from vegetable oils could actually reduce the efficacy of omega-3 PUFAs in fish oil and hence weaken the power of fish oil to reduce cardiovascular disease. These findings appeared to suggest that the presence of excessive vegetable-based omega-6 oils weakens the power of the omega-3 PUFAs derived from fish. Later findings, however, implied that any quantity of fish oil will have some beneficial impact on levels of fats present in the blood, and therefore offer some degree of protection against cardiovascular disease. But remember, optimum benefits will be derived from eating a proper balance between omega-3 and omega-6 PUFAs.

Along with proper diet, the lipid oil extract of the green-lipped mussel can be an important part of achieving this balance. As we have seen, the lipid oil is powerful and efficacious in promoting good health, but it is not a panacea. It must be incorporated into a lifestyle that includes proper nutrition, a regular exercise regimen, and stress reduction.

Now you have been introduced to different types of fatty acids. You know the difference between trans- and cis-fatty acids, and between the omega-6 and the omega-3 groups. You are also familiar with research pointing to the superiority of fish oil in general, and the lipid oil extract of green-lipped mussels in particular. Let's have a closer look at a typical lipid oil capsule. What's in it? And how should you use it?

WHAT'S IN A GREEN-LIPPED MUSSEL LIPID OIL CAPSULE?

An exhaustive catalogue with detailed explanations of all the ingredients in each lipid oil capsule is beyond the purview of this book. In this section, we will review the main ingredients.

Mussel oil. Each lipid oil capsule consists of 50 milligrams of mussel oil. Because pure mussel oil is very sticky and very difficult to handle, it is mixed with 100 milligrams of pharmaceutical-grade olive oil, yielding two parts olive oil and one part lipid oil extract of green-lipped mussels. This may sound like a large quantity of oil but, actually, it's not. In one experiment, patients were given up to fifty capsules of lipid oil extract a day—which equals 5 grams of olive oil, or the equivalent of one small teaspoon. Even as large a dose as fifty capsules of lipid oil a day is not a high-calorie fat item. In fact, this amount is minuscule compared with what we eat normally. When we eat French fries or untrimmed steak, we eat much more fat in a few mouthfuls than we'll find in an entire bottle of green-lipped mussel oil capsules!

Carotenoids. The primary anti-inflammatory agents identified in the lipid oil extract of green-lipped mussels are carotenoids. Carotene is found fairly frequently in fruits and in vegetables such as carrots and dark-leafed greens. The carotenoids are responsible for giving the lipid oil extract its dark orange color. Scientists are still investigating which particular carotenoids are present in the extract. In fact, there has been some speculation that the carotenoids may be unique because so far they have defied exact identification. Certainly, scientists have discovered a wide range of different types of carotenoids in the lipid oil extract of green-lipped mussels. It is probable that they are derived from the plankton that forms the steady diet of the green-lipped mussel.

What do carotenoids do in the body? They are antioxidants. That means they help protect against agents in the blood called free radicals. No, free radicals are not people with bizarre political philosophies who have been let out of jail. They are atoms that bond with various chemical agents, leading to damage caused by oxidation. (Think of what happens when water meets with metal, leading to oxidative rust.) Carotenoids circulate through the body, scavenging for free radicals and protecting against oxidative damage. Some carotenoids, such as beta-carotene, are converted by the body to vitamin A. However, unlike vitamin A supplements, which are toxic if taken in too-high dosages, you cannot overdose on the carotenoids found in the lipid oil extract of green-lipped mussels.

The practical outcomes of this protection are very important and far-reaching. For example, beta-carotene protects patients who are sensitive to sunlight. Every time you soak up the sun, you absorb rays that lead to a damaging oxidative process in your skin. Melanin, the brown pigment responsible for the golden suntan worshipped by Americans, is designed to protect against this photo damage. Too much sun, however, introduces damage beyond the protection that melanin can provide. Antioxidants quench the photo-oxidative process and shield the body from the inflammatory effects of sunburn. But don't go ahead and use lipid oil as sunscreen. It's powerful, but not by itself enough to shield you at the beach—you need all those extra skin-protection factors in sunscreen.

The lipid oil extract of green-lipped mussels and other antioxidants is not only useful in preventing sun-induced skin damage. Free radicals are thought to be partially responsible for skin changes associated with aging. Antioxidants such as beta-carotene may help keep those wrinkles and crow's-feet at bay!

Antioxidant protection is not only skin-deep. Major health conditions can be allayed or prevented by taking antioxidants. A recently published study of more than eighty-nine thousand female nurses from 1980 through 1989 showed that women whose diet included large quantities of vitamin A were less likely to develop breast cancer than women with low intakes of vitamin A—and remember, beta-carotene is converted to vitamin A by the body. As you will see in later chapters of this book, the lipid oil extract's antioxidative effects can be helpful in alleviating a variety of conditions.

A COMPONENT OF GOOD HEALTH

As we have seen, the lipid oil extract of green-lipped mussels is powerful and efficacious in promoting good health. But it's not a panacea. It must be incorporated into a lifestyle that includes proper nutrition, a regular exercise regimen, and stress reduction. We will look at these important elements of a healthy lifestyle later in the book.

Now let's see how the lipid oil extract of green-lipped mussels can address your individual health needs.

3

Joint Disorders and Arthritis

George, 48, owned a garden maintenance and landscaping business. He developed severe, rapidly progressive rheumatoid arthritis. For 14 months, he experienced pain, stiffness, weakness of his hands and wrists, and difficulty walking. He was seriously considering giving up his landscaping business and garden center because he could no longer manage the work or drive his trucks. He was taking a non-steroidal anti-inflammatory drug (NSAID) called naproxen together with aspirin but to no avail. He was in physical pain and was also very depressed.

Then, George began taking four capsules a day of green-lipped mussel oil extract. He did not show up for his follow-up appointment, which was scheduled for a month after his initial appointment. Later, he apologized. He had been outdoors in a blizzard, laying a driveway for a local estate and was so intent on the project that he simply forgot the appointment. He reported that, at first, his symptoms worsened; the hardest day was the third after beginning treatment with the lipid oil. After that, the pain and swelling subsided, his strength improved, and George was able to do all the heavy jobs associated with his business.

Many of you reading this book are seeking relief from the pain and disability associated with arthritis and may be considering the lipid oil extract of green-lipped mussels as a viable option—with good reason. The lipid oil extract's track record in alleviating symptoms of arthritis is excellent. But before we can discuss the role that the lipid oil might play in helping you with your disease, we must first review what arthritis is and how it comes about. It's also important to familiarize yourself with existing self-care and treatment approaches to arthritis and other joint disorders so as to put the lipid oil extract's unique contribution into proper perspective. First, we'll look at the skeletal system and joints and what places them at risk. Then, we'll take a closer look at arthritis, explaining what it is, how it is being approached by doctors today, and how the lipid oil of green-lipped mussels can be helpful.

AN INTRODUCTION TO YOUR JOINTS

We've all seen skeletons—they leer at us on Halloween, they stand in the corners of biology classrooms, and they appear in horror movies. As familiar as we are with what they look like, many of us don't understand exactly what they're made of or what holds them together. The skeleton is the body's supportive framework. It consists mostly of bone, cartilage, and connective tissue. Joints are the connections between any two pieces of skeleton and they enable us to move. Here are the skeleton's functional divisions:

- The skull is primarily a protective bucket turned upside-down over the brain.

- The vertebral column protects the spinal cord and allows freedom of movement. Even more important, it serves as an attachment for the rib cage (the crate that protects the major internal organs), the shoulder and hip girdles, and the appendages (arms and legs) that attach to them. Each appendage (arm or leg) consists of three parts—a large bone closest to the body, one large and one small bone (or one thick and one thin bone) in the middle, and then a number of small bones in the hands or feet.

Flexibility and mobility are the two most important functions of the joints. Imagine a long, hard branch. If you wanted to bend it, you'd have to break it. Now imagine two branches, laid out end to end. In order to form a single unit that can bend into an L, there must be some flexible connection between the two branches. In our bodies, these are called joints.

We often take good joint health for granted. This is a mistake. The strength and resilience of your joints depend on good maintenance. Joints must be used regularly—some of the stiffness you experience when you remain in one position for too long comes from the joint's stiffening up, due to disuse. Physical exercise keeps your joints limber. You also must maintain the strength and health of your bones through engaging in weight-bearing activities. And don't neglect your muscles. Continue to strengthen them through appropriate exercises. All three—muscles, bones, and joints—are part of a total system. For each to remain healthy, the others must also be healthy.

HEALTHY JOINTS: WHAT THEY NEED TO FUNCTION

Healthy bones are hard, strong, and inflexible—which means they don't bend. If you want to wiggle your finger, kneel, or wave your hand, you need flexibility at the point where your bones meet—the joint. Because the bones are hard, bending the area between them might cause them to rub against each other, which would be awkward, painful, and not very efficient. So, your body is supplied with cartilage that serves as a buffer between the bones. Healthy cartilage is also well hydrated and lubricated by synovial fluid to reduce friction when bone surfaces move across each other.

Cartilage is an amazingly versatile material, strong but also springy. It's flexible but won't allow your joints to be bent into destructive positions. Cartilage contains three major components: water, proteoglycans (chemicals consisting primarily of a protein core), and collagen, another agent produced by the body. Collagen is the most important component of cartilage and is responsible for maintaining its structural integrity. However, the proteoglycans are also critical. They contain additional components—including glycosaminoglycan, chondroitin sulfate, and keratin sulfate—that are currently under investigation in regard to arthritis.

WHAT PLACES JOINTS AT RISK?

Arguments have abounded among scientists for centuries regarding "nature versus nurture." Are we formed primarily by inborn, genetic factors or by environmental factors? Today's scientists believe that this dichotomy is too simplistic and that the answer to this question isn't black-and-white. Rather, a mixture of genetic and environmental factors contributes to most illnesses. Joint diseases are no exception: people with genetic tendencies toward joint disorders are more vulnerable to environmental insults; conversely, people who continually abuse their joints may develop injury-induced disorders, even if such conditions do not run in their families.

Let's look at risk factors for joint disorders—circumstances and conditions that raise the risk of falling victim to diseases of the joints—as well as suggest some solutions to minimize the potential damage.

Genetic Factors

While scientists have not yet identified the specific genes responsible for the development of joint disorders, especially osteoarthritis (OA), it is known that these conditions tend to run in families. If you have a family history of OA, you may develop the disorder as a result of the normal aging process, even if you protect your joints. It is likely that the first signs will appear after the age of fifty-five. If you have been involved with sports, you may develop symptoms sooner.

When I use the word *symptoms,* I don't necessarily mean excruciating pain, swelling, or inflammation. Some people have joints that are stressed and damaged, but are not inflamed. These people do not suffer from pain or great discomfort. Others have relatively minor signs of joint damage—at least based on the evidence of X-rays and biopsies—but have a great deal of inflammation. These individuals suffer greatly. And many people have damage that falls between the two extremes.

If arthritis runs in your family, it is imperative that you become involved in a joint-protection program as early as possible. Ideally, you should begin to take measures to shield your joints from injury while you are in your teens. But, obviously, you can't turn back the clock if you're older. You can, however, teach your own children how to protect their joints. And at whatever stage in life you find yourself, you can begin to care for your joints now.

Sports

Sports play a big role in the long-term progression of OA. Scientists have focused a great deal of attention on people involved in sports, studying the impact of athletic activities on the joints. Professional athletes, college students who are intensely involved in sports, and people who regularly engage in a sport as a hobby are all vulnerable to sport-induced injuries. By the term *injuries,* I don't necessarily mean broken arms and sprained ankles; rather, I'm talking about a more subtle process—the damage done by years of straining the same set of joints.

For example, you may have developed a style of running—a particular set of motions you use to place one foot in front of the other—or you may have developed an especially powerful tennis serve that knocks your opponent cold every time. Insofar as these moves "work," you feel that they are functional—you do, after all, manage to run to your destination or hit the tennis ball into your opponent's court. And as long as you don't limp off the track or the court with serious injuries, you also feel that you're doing no harm to yourself. But actually, you may be inflicting subtle insults upon your joints with every competition. You may have learned a series of moves or techniques that stress your joints and cause long-term damage.

It's easy to disregard the notion of an injury that develops over time, a process that creeps up on you as you age. Most twenty-five year olds probably think themselves to be virtually invulnerable to the slow deteriorative process of aging. Athletes are particularly notorious for disregarding the wear and tear put on their bodies by their physical activities. Precisely because of their physical prowess, they think of themselves as being above the normal physiological processes that affect the rest of us mortals. The result: they do severe damage to their joints. I have seen thirty-five year olds with crippling OA induced by irresponsible athletic activities such as the repeated use of shoes with poor support or inadequate cushioning. These patients, who should be in the prime of their physical lives, are invalids.

There is also a series of destructive beliefs that abound among athletes, many of whom are subjected to extreme peer pressure to internalize and act on those beliefs. One of the most destructive attitudes is "no pain, no gain"—the belief that without experiencing pain, their exercise is worthless. For some athletes, this philosophy is carried to the point of masochism. Remember that pain is an important signal, your body's way of informing you that something is wrong. It waves a red flag in front of your face, begging you to stop whatever activity is causing the pain.

Pain should be responded to not only by discontinuing the offending activity, but also by taking some type of medication that will alleviate it. As far back as the 1920s, studies showed that if the sensation of pain is stopped by injecting an anesthetic at the trunk of the affected nerve, inflammation at the end of the nerve is also prevented. The anesthetic is not in and of itself an anti-inflammatory agent. Rather, the pain seems to release inflammatory substances, so by blocking the pain, you also block the release of these substances. Painkillers such as acetaminophen are not anti-inflammatory in action, but can nevertheless be helpful for those suffering from arthritis, because they help to break the vicious cycle of inflammation. A study published in the *New England Journal of Medicine* showed that acetaminophen is as effective as an NSAID for most people who suffer from osteoarthritis. While excessive doses can lead to liver damage, ordinary doses are free from side effects.

Joint protection can be accomplished by taking a responsible approach to sports. Always be sure you receive proper coaching and training. A good coach isn't necessarily the person who knows the best strategies to stymie the opposing football team. A good coach will know the best strategies to protect your joints from injury. This is even more important than winning the game. You will have to live with your joints long after the applause and fanfare have died down. Whether you will be able to run, walk, or even sit without pain will depend on how you protect your joints during your athletic years.

With the assistance of your trainer or coach, you can observe your exercise style. Do you run heel first or toe first? Do your feet come down on their sides? You can purchase special inserts for your athletic shoes, depending on where your feet fall when you run. These serve as shock absorbers, cushioning your feet from the repetitive blows that take place every time they meet the concrete. Minimizing shock is very important. Obviously, if you play basketball, you're unlikely to be pounding your feet against concrete, but if you're a runner, try to choose a soft surface like a dirt track rather than a hard concrete track. And always make sure your footwear is in good shape to provide maximum cushioning.

Microtraumas

Microtraumas are tiny traumas: each one may not be powerful enough to cause injury, but a series of these traumas can eventually cause a great deal of damage. Imagine a rock with water dripping on it. Each drop of water has no impact on the rock, but a steady trickle of droplets over enough time will erode the rock and eventually make a hole in it.

For example, leaping out of bed in the morning places daily stress on the joints. If you tend to oversleep, then catapult yourself into your clothes, you are not giving your joints enough time to become lubricated after a period of relative immobility during the night. Many alarm clocks come with a "snooze" button. If you set your alarm to go off a few minutes before you actually need to get up, you can get the rust out of your joints while moving slowly in bed. By the time you *really* need to get up, you have begun the lubricative process and protected your joints from assault.

There are a variety of professions that involve physical activities that "drip-drip" steadily until joints have been damaged. People who stand on their feet all day, such as hairdressers, dentists, sales clerks, airline attendants, or waiters, put a great deal of weight on their hips, knees, and ankles. People who engage in repetitive activities that involve the knees, hips, hands, elbows, or shoulders may develop arthritis, especially if they are subjected to vibrations, such as people who work on a conveyer belt at a factory or are involved in repairing machinery. Certainly construction workers and others who engage in repetitive lifting and lugging of heavy objects place their joints at risk.

Here, too, you need to take careful note of your lifestyle. Are you a door-to-door letter carrier? You will need shoes that support your feet for the type of walking you do. Are you a waiter who does a lot of standing (while taking orders) and then walking (to and from the kitchen)? You may need to purchase footwear that is designed for these types of activities. Specialized shoe stores often have computers that can help you find a shoe that fits your feet and your activities.

If you work at a computer, with your wrists immobilized for long periods of time while typing on the keyboard, or if you perform other repetitive work, you will need to remind yourself to take frequent breaks. Some mild stretching exercises may offset some of the damaging effects of these repetitive motions. You may need to fight for your right to do this on the job, but I encourage you to do so. Employers are becoming increasingly aware of work-induced injuries. It is in their best interests to provide the most health-enhancing work environment for their employees, so as to cut down on sick time and to avoid legal action in the event of injury.

Imbalanced Legs

It may sound strange to you, but your legs probably are not completely symmetrical. This doesn't mean that you look grotesquely lopsided, but simply that, for most people, one leg is almost always just a little longer than the other. And the difference between the legs rarely remains constant, because at a certain point we stop growing. We grow until the age of twenty-five, after which we start to lose height. Rarely does this process balance out the legs. More often, it accentuates the difference. So, if you want to protect your hips, spine, and knees from wear and tear induced by imbalance, it's important to balance your legs on a regular basis. An orthopedist or podiatrist can measure the distance between your heel and the crest of your iliac bone. It's important to be assessed by a professional because just fractions of millimeters of difference can have a consequence over the long term. You can maintain the balance of your legs by inserting and wearing an appropriate inner sole.

Environmental Factors

Arthritis is aggravated by cold, damp environments. England and Scandinavia, both with cold, damp climates, are known for their high rates of arthritis. Whether or not you have a family history of arthritis, make sure you keep yourself warm and dry at all times. Don't lie around in a wet bathing suit; change into dry clothes as soon as possible. Take an extra sweater or scarf wherever you go in case the weather turns unexpectedly chilly. Make sure your bed-covers are thick and cozy, and sleep in a warm room so if you uncover yourself during the night, you won't get chilled.

Nutritional Factors

Although we discussed nutrition in detail in Chapter 2, it is worth touching on a few of the points again because they are so important. First, the strong preponderance of trans-fatty acids as well as omega-6 oils in our diet sets us up for inflammation. The omega-6 group increases the supply of arachidonic acid, the precursor of prostaglandins, thromboxanes, leukotrienes, and other mediators of inflammation. Individuals living in southern Greece, for example, have a very low incidence of rheumatoid arthritis because they eat large quantities of cooked vegetables and use primarily olive oil, a natural source of monounsaturated fatty acids (MUFAs), which do not stimulate inflammation.

Interestingly, the French also have a lower incidence of joint disorders, even though they don't eat large quantities of fish oil or consume lots of omega-3 oils, such as flaxseed, or borage. Scientists refer to this as the "French paradox." It may be that duck, goose, and chicken fats—staples of the French diet—are actually rich in monounsaturated fatty acids. Even butter and cream, when eaten raw, do not necessarily have deleterious effects on the joints. It is the heating of these fats that causes them to become oxidized, with all their destructive results.

If you want to protect your joints, you must begin to make some dietary changes. These will be helpful not only for your joints but also for your cardiovascular system, as we'll see in the next chapter. They are recommended for everyone, and they are imperative for individuals with a family history of arthritis.

Obesity

Obesity is not merely a cosmetic problem but a medical problem as well, and it has reached almost epidemic proportions in most Western countries. Being overweight puts strain and pressure on joints, even when you're lying down. After all, the horizontal position does not suppress gravity. If we were not subject to the laws of gravity even while lying down, we'd float into space at bedtime. So the pressure on our bones and joints is real, even if there is no vertical gravity involved.

When you're standing, the pressure on joints rises, because the joints must lug around heavier and heavier loads. The combination of overeating, guzzling soft drinks like colas, and living a sedentary lifestyle contribute to obesity. For example, it has been thoroughly documented that young girls who watch too much television and eat excessively large quantities of fattening foods are more likely to be obese and to develop arthritic conditions at an early age—especially in their hips and knees, which are the joints that must carry the extra weight. Arthritis doesn't confine itself to overweight individuals, but obesity certainly increases the risk.

Stress

Most of us experience stress at one point or other in our lives. I'm not just talking about major psychological traumas—death, illness of a loved one, job loss, or divorce. Even the "minor" day-to-day

glitches and difficulties (schedules too tightly packed, unantici-
pated workload, a plumber who doesn't show up) are stressful.

There is evidence that people who are under stress have an
unconscious tendency to contract their muscles. Tension headaches, for example, are caused by the tightening up of neck muscles. Fibromyalgia, a chronic pain syndrome identified relatively
recently, is associated with tension in the neck and back muscles
that leads to pain. So, psychological stress doesn't confine itself to
the mind but also affects the muscles. Tense, contracted muscles, in
turn, have a negative impact on the joints because it is harder for
bones to move freely when muscles are contracted. The muscle
spasm constricts the joint and, over time, can cause damage.

Techniques such as yoga, biofeedback, meditation, relaxation,
and visualization that relieve psychological stress can also provide
relief for the physical stress. This improves and reduces the inflammation associated with joint damage.

*Mary, 41, was initially diagnosed with rheumatoid arthritis. She started
to feel unwell approximately one year prior to being seen and she developed increasing stiffness and felt she was aging rapidly. Mary suffered
from severe fatigue and pronounced weakness of the arms and hands. She
woke up in the morning feeling stiff and remained so all day. She had difficulty both bending down and climbing stairs.*

*Prior to the illness, she had been very active. One of her favorite
activities had been horseback riding, but for several months, she had been
unable to ride. She was very despondent because she missed her horse. The
ibuprofen that she was taking upset her stomach and did little to alleviate the pain and stiffness. Her saliva and tears had dried up during the
course of the illness, so she was also taking artificial saliva and tears.*

*Two weeks after starting on green-lipped mussel oil extract (four cap-
sules per day), she felt much better. Her stiffness and pain were gone, and
her strength had returned; so had her tears and saliva. She had much
more energy and had started to ride her horse again. One week later, she
was riding with ease.*

*She has continued to do well and has no problems with her joints,
eyes, or saliva as long as she continues to take the lipid oil. When she for-
gets or runs out of the oil, the symptoms return but are reversed rapidly*

when she recommences taking the oil extract. She no longer needs any NSAIDs or artificial tears or saliva.

HOW INFLAMMATION DAMAGES JOINTS

Before we can understand the unique contribution the lipid oil of green-lipped mussels can make to the treatment of arthritis, we must first understand what arthritis is and how doctors currently approach it.

Damage to joints causes inflammation to both the joints and their adjacent tissues—inflammation that leads to pain, stiffness, joint enlargement, and more inflammation. What is inflammation anyway? When you sustain an injury or when an alien organism (virus, fungus, or bacterium) invades, the body responds by releasing a series of chemicals, which can cause redness, swelling, pain, and impeded function. Strange as this may sound, these are actually desirable bodily responses, as unpleasant as they may be. They are the body's way of protecting you against infection.

Injury damages the integrity of the skin as well as connective tissue, muscle, and blood vessels. This places you at risk of infection, which can be caused by the entry of harmful organisms through the ruptured and damaged surface. The body must respond to injury by repairing and healing the damaged tissue. To do so, the blood vessels expand to transport more chemicals to the affected area. The tiny blood vessels—the capillaries—become more permeable: the usually tight, protective blood-vessel walls relax to allow larger molecules of invasion fighters out to do "battle" with the invading organism or help repair the damaged site. Finally, chemicals leave the capillaries and enter surrounding tissues.

Among the many powerful chemicals released by the capillaries are leukotrienes, which we discussed in detail in Chapter 2. Leukotrienes are produced by the LOX pathway, while the COX pathway releases other inflammatory substances called prostaglandins and thromboxanes. Each plays a different role in creating inflammation.

In autoimmune diseases, such as arthritis and asthma, the

body reacts by calling in the equivalent of the National Guard, as if there were a foreign invader, when in reality none is present. Of course, after the discussion of risk factors, you can understand that in reality there is a small but steady stream of "microinvaders"— mini-insults causing minor, undetectable inflammatory responses that eventually build up over time to create a state of chronic inflammation. It is as if the soldiers "set up camp" at a particular site and never leave, because they continue to "expect" an invasion to occur.

There are two types of arthritis—osteoarthritis (OA) and rheumatoid arthritis (RA). While the inflammatory process occurring in each may be similar, and microtraumas may play an important role in both conditions, osteoarthritis is more frequently caused by "impact injury" or the "wear and tear" of life. OA more commonly creeps up with the onset of older age. Rheumatoid arthritis, on the other hand, is strictly an autoimmune disorder. While it may be exacerbated by serious or minor injury, it is not caused by these factors. Ultimately, scientists are still struggling to understand why the body suddenly "decides" to turn against itself in autoimmune disorders.

Both types of arthritis seem to have their chemical origins right in the affected joints. It has been discovered that joints contain mast cells, which play an important role in the inflammatory process. When activated, they release inflammatory mediators associated with inflammation—histamine, leukotrienes, prostaglandins, and thromboxanes. Uncovering the role of mast cells in inflammation represents an important scientific discovery because it demonstrates that inflammation in the joints is not imported from elsewhere in the body, but originates in the joints themselves. This makes joints even more vulnerable than previously thought to the steady onslaught of microtraumas and other injuries.

ARTHRITIS AND INFLAMMATION

Arthritis does its damage by causing inflammation to the joints and adjacent tissues. This inflammation leads to pain, stiffness, cracking, joint enlargement, and, in turn, more inflammation. In fact, the word "arthritis" means "joint inflammation." It is a catchall term, however, referring to a group of more than 100 rheumatic diseases that can cause pain, stiffness, and swelling in the joints. These diseases may affect not only the joints but also other parts of the body, including important supporting structures such as muscles, bones, tendons, and ligaments, as well as some internal organs.

Up to 50 million Americans—one in seven people—may suffer from arthritis, and almost everyone over the age of fifty has signs of it. Although arthritis can affect people in the prime of their lives (almost 9 million adults), there is a higher prevalence in elderly individuals. Women are more likely than men to suffer from arthritis and, in fact, arthritis is the most prevalent chronic condition in women, affecting nearly 23 million.

Whether you're male or female, you are at serious risk of disability if you suffer from arthritis, which is the leading cause of disability in America. It causes limitations of activity in approximately 7 million Americans. That means it causes more disability than heart and lung conditions, diabetes, or even cancer. These are disturbing and sobering figures and it is not an exaggeration to say that arthritis is a national emergency.

When you see an elderly person hobbling along, painfully leaning on a cane, you can assume the person probably is suffering from some form or arthritis. Movement is difficult, labored, and painful. The fingers move slowly, the legs no longer appear to obey the person's commands. Inflammation has run amok and is causing serious damage to mobility. As modern medicine continues to find new and exciting ways to prolong life, and the population of senior citizens continues to rise, we will see an increasing number of older adults who cannot enjoy the gift of long life to its fullest.

TYPES OF ARTHRITIS

We've touched briefly on the distinction between the two types of arthritis, osteoarthritis (OA) and rheumatoid arthritis (RA). While they may have some similar symptoms and, certainly, both are caused by inflammation, they have a different cause and also affect different parts of the body.

Rheumatologists look at two pairs of major joints, the knees and the hips, for the diagnosis of osteoarthritis. With gout and rheumatoid arthritis, the small joints, such as those in the hands (with gout, the toes) are mainly affected, although large joints can also be involved. Many more people are affected with OA because it's associated with aging and trauma; RA and gout, on the other hand, have a stronger genetic component.

Osteoarthritis

Osteoarthritis is often called "wear and tear" arthritis because it is usually caused by the impact of a prolonged series of microtraumas associated with the normal process of daily life, rather than with an autoimmune disorder. There are at least twenty-five different forms of OA. Although it can occur in people under the age of forty-five, OA most often occurs with the onset of one's fifties and sixties. It is a slow and progressive condition that generally affects the weight-bearing joints of the knees and hips, as well as the lower back, neck, and fingers.

While the inflammation in OA comes from several different locations in and around the bone, cartilage breakdown is its main feature. Inflammatory mediators are increased in the damaged cartilage. Additionally, the surrounding fluid—called synovial fluid—also exudes some inflammatory substances, including matrix metalloproteinases, collagenases, and prostaglandins. Together with other chemical agents, these degrade the collagen and proteoglycans present in healthy cartilage. Nitrous oxide production increases and a process called apoptosis occurs. *Apoptosis* means "programmed cell death" and it happens when cells self-destruct because they have become too damaged to survive and to replicate into new, healthy cells. As OA progresses, more cartilage is degraded, and the mechanics of joint use change, creating additional irritation, which further promotes inflammation; and so the process continues and the condition worsens.

OA can take many different forms. For example, chondritis occurs when chondrocytes—the cartilage cells responsible for producing the building blocks of healthy cartilage—synthesize prostaglandins, which are inflammatory chemicals. Chondrocytes do this in response to cytokines, which are messenger proteins that enable cells to influence one another. Cytokines are not by any means undesirable substances—they are an important aspect of the body's immune system. However, in osteoarthritis, they are "overmessaging" and "calling in the troops" inappropriately, which leads to further joint damage and inflammation.

Osteitis occurs when the damage spreads to the bone, and synovitis occurs when the synovial lining tissue—the membrane located on the interface between the cartilage and the bone—becomes inflamed. Synovitis occurs frequently with OA, and the degree of inflammation predicts the response to non-steroidal anti-inflammatory drugs (NSAIDs).

Rheumatoid Arthritis

Rheumatoid arthritis, which is an autoimmune disorder, is a crippling disease that affects about 2.1 million Americans, or about 1% of the population, most of them women. While RA is not itself fatal, sufferers are at increased risk for other illnesses, such as adult-onset diabetes and gastrointestinal bleeding. These illnesses shorten life spans by an average of between five and fifteen years.

There are at least ninety different forms of RA and their causes are not fully understood. It can be triggered by environmental factors, a bacterial or viral infection, stress, and even hormonal imbalances following pregnancy. Although it is aggravated by injury, RA is ultimately due to a mysterious disease process that is probably genetic in origin. While a competent rheumatologist should make the diagnosis, you can guess at which condition you have based on your symptoms. RA generally is characterized by symmetrical joint swelling—the corresponding joints on both sides of the body are likely to be affected. You may experience pain and swelling in the second and third knuckles and middle joints of both hands, for example. The balls of your toes may become painful. And you may experience extended stiffness upon awakening in the morning.

Your doctor will look for swelling and thickening in the synovial lining (the lining of the joints). He or she may order laboratory tests to ascertain whether your blood shows elevated markers of inflammation. Over 75% of patients with RA test positive for rheumatoid factor in the blood. Your doctor may also order X-rays to ascertain whether there is evidence of a narrowing in the joint space.

RA can also spread to internal organs. The inflammation can move to the internal lining of the lungs (a condition called pleurisy) or to the peripheral nerves. When this happens, you may experience numbness or tingling from neuropathy. You need to be on the alert for anemia, because RA can affect the bone marrow, which is an important component in producing red blood cells. Your eyes and even the lining of your heart may be affected. So if you have RA, it's vital to place yourself under the care of a rheumatologist who will take regular blood tests to measure your levels of rheumatoid factor. These will provide important clues as to your vulnerability to the spread of inflammation.

Bonita, 43, thought she was suffering from arthritis, which ran in her family. Although the diagnosis had never been confirmed, her shoulders were often stiff and painful, especially on awakening and before a rainstorm. She also suffered from fibromyalgia and constant neck and head pain due to two herniated discs at the base of her scalp.

Bonita was unable to take ibuprofen for the pain because of its negative effects on the stomach coupled with her history of ulcers. She tried using acetaminophen, but her headaches continued to worsen and began to affect her work and her relationships.

Bonita heard about green-lipped mussel oil extract through a friend and began using it to alleviate the symptoms of arthritis. She knew that there was no risk in trying the mussel oil because it has no negative side effects. Within two weeks, the pain in her shoulders had completely disappeared. She also found, to her amazement, that many of her other symptoms had resolved—her neck pain became almost negligible, the general fibromyalgia-induced achiness throughout her body disappeared, and she has not had a single headache since starting the lipid oil.

TREATMENT OPTIONS FOR ARTHRITIS

It's time for a thorough review of available treatment options for arthritis. Some of these therapies offer only short-term relief, while others boast longer-term results.

Painkillers

There are several categories of painkillers—each works somewhat differently in the body, with its own set of properties and side effects. Non-steroidal anti-inflammatory drugs (NSAIDs) like aspirin and ibuprofen, for example, are painkillers with anti-inflammatory benefits as well. Unfortunately, they also have serious side effects, such as digestive disturbances, gastritis, esophagitis, and bleeding ulcers. Some people develop even more serious problems, such as kidney failure or hemorrhage in the brain. While these medications can in all fairness be considered miracle drugs because they help millions of people to experience relief from relentless pain, their side effects have been extremely problematic.

Acetaminophen is an effective painkiller, although it does not have anti-inflammatory properties. However, when used over an extended period of time, it can have a negative impact on the liver. You can use NSAIDs and acetaminophen to obtain short-term relief when you have a flare-up of arthritic symptoms, but for more chronic problems, you need to look for other solutions because of the side effects associated with long-term use.

Corticosteroids

Corticosteroids are hormones, taken by mouth or given by injection, that are very effective in treating arthritis. Prednisone is the corticosteroid most often used orally to reduce the inflammation associated with RA. However, oral steroids have an array of severe side effects. Corticosteroids can also be injected directly into a joint to stop pain. Frequent injections may damage the cartilage and should only be used once or twice a year.

COX-2 Inhibitors

In 1999, drug manufacturers introduced a class of NSAIDs called COX-2 inhibitors (sometimes called COX-2 selective inhibitors). The drugs were bestsellers from the start. Arthritis sufferers were eager to take medications that eased joint pain without causing gastrointestinal pain, bleeding, and other side effects. In the year after their introduction, doctors wrote over 100 million prescriptions for celecoxib (Celebrex) and rofecoxib (Vioxx). Celebrex is now the sixth bestselling drug, with sales of more than $4 billion since its debut in 1999; Vioxx had sales amounting to $2.6 billion in 2001.

The idea behind COX-2 inhibitors is to offer people with arthritis the benefits of NSAIDs without the harmful side effects. NSAIDs work by halting the production of prostaglandins, and to do that, they interrupt the activity of COX-1 and COX-2 enzymes. Most of the harmful side effects of NSAIDs result from the interruption of COX-1 enzymes, which help produce the mucus in the stomach lining that protects against ulcers. COX-2 inhibitors are supposed to only inhibit the COX-2 enzymes that bring about pain and inflammation; they leave the COX-1 enzymes involved in stomach mucus production alone.

In theory they only inhibit COX-2 enzymes, but in practice, the jury is still deliberating. COX-2 inhibitors may erode the stomach's mucus protection, although the drugs are not supposed to be as harmful to the gastrointestinal tract as other NSAIDs. Like other NSAIDs, the drugs may damage the kidneys. But more importantly, COX-2 inhibitors significantly increase the risk of heart attacks and strokes. Others have called into question the drugs' benefits given how expensive they are compared to other NSAIDs. COX-2 inhibitors cost roughly $2.75 per tablet, significantly more than naproxen, for example, which costs 18 cents.

Much to the displeasure of pharmaceutical giants Pfizer and Merck, the makers of Celebrex and Vioxx, respectively, the Food and Drug Administration (FDA) requires COX-2 inhibitor drugs to carry the same gastrointestinal risk warning as other NSAIDs. In February 2000, on the strength of new studies they had commissioned, Pharmacia (which merged with Pfizer in 2003) and Merck asked the Arthritis Advisory Committee to the FDA to review whether these warnings were necessary. The Committee concluded that the studies did not show that COX-2 inhibitors have a "clinically meaningful" safety advantage over standard NSAIDs, nor did they show an overall reduction in gastrointestinal complications. The gastrointestinal health warnings remain on the labels of COX-2 inhibitors.

NSAIDs decrease blood flow to the kidneys, and for that reason, they have been linked to kidney failure, especially in elderly patients and patients with pre-existing kidney damage. COX-2 inhibitors, it appears, are no different from other NSAIDs in their affect on the kidneys. In a study published in the *Annals of Internal Medicine* (July 4, 2000), researchers had 75 patients aged sixty to eighty years with normally functioning kidneys take the COX-2 inhibitor rofecoxib (Vioxx), the NSAID indomethacin (Indocid, Novo-Methacin), or a placebo. Subjects in all three groups were placed on a low-sodium diet because salt intake can affect test results in kidney studies. In groups taking the COX-2 inhibitor and the NSAID, the subjects' ability to filter waste products declined to the same degree. In other words, COX-2 inhibitors are as likely as standard NSAIDs to cause problems for the kidneys.

Another troubling aspect of COX-2 inhibitors is the drugs' potential to increase the risk of heart attacks and strokes. In 2001, cardiologists at the Cleveland Clinic analyzed clinical trials of COX-2 inhibitors to determine if these drugs have any affect on cardiovascular health. In a trial involving 8,059 people with rheumatoid arthritis who were given the COX-2 inhibitor rofecoxib (Vioxx) or the NSAID diclofenac, patients taking the COX-2 inhibitor were twice as likely to have a heart attack, stroke, or other cardiovascular event. This trial was supposed to exclude people who had a history of heart disease, but 321 subjects with heart disease were included in the study by mistake. Among these people, patients who took the COX-2 inhibitor were four times more likely to have a cardiovascular event. This trial was significant because the subjects weren't permitted to take aspirin, a drug known to protect against heart attacks. The Cleveland Clinic also looked at a trial involving roughly 8,000 patients who took celecoxib (Celebrex) or an NSAID. Patients were allowed to take aspirin during this trial. The trial revealed no difference in cardiovascular events between the group taking COX-2 inhibitors and the group taking standard NSAIDs, but this may have been attributable to the patients' taking aspirin, according to the Cleveland Clinic.

Neither trial that the Cleveland Clinic analyzed was initially designed to investigate cardiovascular events (they were designed to compare the effect of COX-2 inhibitors and NSAIDs on the gastrointestinal tract). Moreover, although the drugs double the risk of getting a heart attack, the risk remains quite low. Still, these trials raise concerns because they point to something in COX-2 inhibitors that can cause heart disease. As early as 1999, the National Academy of Sciences warned that COX-2 inhibitors increase the risk of strokes, heart attacks, and blood-clotting disorders. One theory is that they suppress the production of a prostaglandin called prostacyclin in the walls of blood vessels that acts to dilate the vessels and inhibit blood clots. So concerned is the FDA that COX-2 inhibitors increase the risk of heart attacks, the agency's Health and Human Services Department cited Merck (the maker of Vioxx) in a September 21, 2001 warning letter. Merck, the agency wrote, has "engaged in a promotional campaign for Vioxx that minimizes the potentially serious cardiovascular findings that were observed . . . and thus, misrepresents the safety profile for Vioxx."

Finally, the high cost of COX-2 inhibitors relative to other NSAIDs has caused some to question whether the drugs are cost-effective. In some studies, the absolute risk reduction of taking COX-2 inhibitors is only 1% or 2% compared to other NSAIDs. If the risk reduction is this low, is spending an extra $500 to $700 a year for COX-2 inhibitors worthwhile? To measure the cost-effectiveness of COX-2 inhibitors, researchers at the University of California at Los Angeles and the V.A. Greater Los Angeles Healthcare System devised a quality-adjusted life-year measurement scale for a hypothetical sixty-year-old patient with mild to severe arthritic pain. The study found that COX-2 inhibitors cost $275,809 more than naproxen to produce each additional life-year; for patients with heart disease, COX-2 inhibitors cost $395,324 more. The authors concluded: "The risk reduction seen with coxibs (COX-2 inhibitors) does not offset their increased costs compared with nonselective NSAIDs in the management of average-risk patients with chronic arthritis. However, coxibs may provide an acceptable incremental cost-effectiveness ratio in the subgroup of patients with a history of bleeding ulcers."

Some have suggested that COX-2 inhibitors were placed on the market before sufficient studies were done as to their effectiveness and that the drugs were pushed too hard and too fast by pharmaceutical companies. Larry Sasich, a pharmacist for the Public Citizen Health Research Group, put it this way: "The question prescribers have to ask is how did Celebrex reach $1 billion in sales at a time when there wasn't a single controlled trial published that looked at the effectiveness in treating arthritis and pain compared to similar drugs. What sources of information do prescribers use to choose drugs? In the case of Celebrex, because there was no science, the decision had to be based on promotional materials." In the fall of 2004, Merck withdrew Vioxx from all markets, and is facing 140,000 lawsuits from families of patients who suffered heart attacks attributable to Vioxx. Another COX-2 inhibitor, valdecoxib (Bextra), manufactured by Pfizer, was also withdrawn from the market in 2005 at the request of the FDA because of cardiovascular safety concerns.

Cyclosporin

A potent suppressor of the immune system, cyclosporin may be indicated in severe cases that are either life-threatening or completely crippling. Because suppressing the immune system can have such serious side effects, cyclosporin should be used only as a last-resort approach.

Antirheumatic Drugs

Antirheumatic drugs are used to treat people with RA who have not responded to NSAIDs. Some of these medications are methotrexate, hydroxychloroquine, penicillamine, and gold injections. Recently, monoclonal antibodies have been studied, and some have received FDA approval. These drugs are thought to influence and correct abnormalities of the immune system responsible for a disease like RA. Treatment with these medications requires careful monitoring by a physician to avoid side effects.

Surgery

Two types of surgery are used to address arthritis—palliative surgery, which is designed to alleviate pain, and replacement surgery, which replaces damaged joints with artificial alternatives. A surgeon may remove the synovium, realign the joint, or even replace the damaged joint with an artificial one. Total joint replacement has provided not only dramatic relief from pain, but also improvement in motion.

Proper Diet

If you want to protect your joints, you must make some dietary changes. These will be helpful not only for your joints but also for your cardiovascular system. They are recommended for everyone, but they are imperative for individuals with a family history of arthritis.

- Switch to MUFA-rich vegetable oils, such as canola and olive oil.

- Many animal fats that are consumed in small amounts carry MUFAs: foie gras, chicken fat, and raw butter are certainly healthier than margarine or other hydrogenated "spreads." However, you should avoid organ meats, red meats, and egg yolks because they are high in the type of fats that store arachidonic acid.

  If you must have red meat or eggs, choose range-fed cattle and wild game, and eggs from free-range chickens. These tend to be lower in fat, and the fat they do contain is usually lower in arachidonic acid. Trim as much visible fat as possible from your steaks. Try grilling rather than frying, and marinate your red meat in a mixture of one cup of red wine and one cup of olive or light sesame oil for twenty-four hours. Drain, season, and grill. The wine leaches out a fair amount of saturated fat in the steak, and the olive oil replaces it with monounsaturated fat. Make omelets from two egg whites per one egg yolk. You can scramble your eggs with ricotta cheese or tofu to add consistency and flavor. Experiment with removing egg yolks from other recipes.

- Avoid cookies, crackers, and foods processed with "hydrogenated" oils as they contain trans-fatty acids.

- Increase your consumption of fish, such as salmon, mackerel, and other seafood that is high in fat. They are high in omega-3 polyunsaturated fatty acids (PUFAs). However, if you don't like fish or are allergic to it, you can obtain these PUFAs from vegetable oils. And you can supplement with a high-quality marine-oil supplement such as green-lipped mussel oil.

- Saturated fat shouldn't be rejected entirely. Coconut and palm oils demonstrate powerful antioxidant properties that offset their potential danger as "rich in saturated fats." The key is balance.

- Balance your fats. Your ratio of omega-6 to omega-3 PUFAs should be 1:1 or 2:1. That means you should be eating, at most, twice as much omega-6 as omega-3 PUFAs. Monounsaturated fats are also acceptable.

- Limit your fats. A good diet should provide less than 2,000 calories a day. You should keep your fat intake to less than 20% of your total caloric intake, with trans-fatty acids kept to a minimum. Sure, enjoy a plate of French fries or a few cookies from time to time, but be sure you keep your quantities small and your intake very occasional.

- Good nutrition doesn't only involve oils—you need a well-balanced diet with enough protein, vegetables, vitamins, and minerals. You also need fiber. Processed foods are notoriously low in fiber and in important minerals, such as magnesium. Magnesium is an important mineral for those who want to prevent arthritis or to reduce its symptoms. Good sources of magnesium include traditional hearty breads, whole-wheat pasta, legumes, dried fruits, nuts, and some mineral waters.

• Remember to drink plenty of water. People who have a tendency for arthritis have even more need for water than others. Why? Because water is an essential component of healthy cartilage and necessary for lubrication of the area between the joints. While coffee, tea, alcohol, and soft drinks all provide liquid, water is best because it flushes out impurities and toxins in the joints instead of adding more. How much water should you drink? A quick way to figure your water intake is to divide your body weight in half; that's how many ounces of water you need to absorb each day to flush toxins out of your joints. You don't have to have it all in the form of fluids—remember that there is water in many foods as well.

• Avoid chili peppers. Capsaicin, an active ingredient in chili peppers, releases a chemical called Substance P that creates inflammation around nerve endings. It will aggravate an inflammatory process if it runs in your family.

Your diet is a crucial aspect of your overall health and is very important in helping you prevent arthritis and reduce the symptoms if you already suffer from it.

Weight Reduction

Excess pounds put extra stress on weight-bearing joints such as the knees or hips. Studies have shown that overweight women who lost an average of eleven pounds substantially reduced the development of OA in their knees. In addition, if OA has already affected one knee, you can protect the other knee by removing weight-induced stress.

Exercise

Exercise builds muscle strength and also relieves psychological stress. I'm not talking here about sports activities, but rather about aerobic exercise as well as strength-building exercises such as weight lifting. As with any physical activity, there is the potential of injury, so it's important to check with an exercise therapist, coach, or trainer before embarking upon an exercise program. You must make sure you are not engaging in repetitive motions that will ultimately cause more stress than they alleviate. You should also be checked over by your physician, especially if you're over the age of forty-five, to make sure you have a clean bill of health before exercising. If you are experiencing some type of health problem, you may need specialized advice about how to exercise safely.

Safe exercise has enormous benefits for your joints as well as your psyche. Here's an activity that might relieve both psychological and physical stress—and involves a certain amount of physical exercise and activity. I'm referring to sex. People who enjoy a happy sex life tend to have less stress and less pain. It is well documented that orgasms, especially in women, produce some analgesia that relieves pain. There can also be a great release of tension in the orgasm—not to mention the additional emotional benefits of intimacy, support, and companionship that are so important if you are going through a difficult time. Find a way to incorporate this wonderful and natural stress-reducer into your life on a more frequent basis.

Swimming, walking, low-impact aerobic exercise, and range-of-motion exercises may reduce joint pain and stiffness. In addition, stretching exercises such as yoga are helpful.

Glucosamine

Glucosamine is a chondro-protective agent, providing the body with the raw materials to regenerate cartilage necessary for healthy joint function. In order for OA to be treated effectively, the cartilage and synovial fluid in the joint must be protected against further destruction. At the same time, it is desirable to stimulate restoration of joint cartilage and synovial fluid. Research seems to indicate that chondro-protective agents protect and restore joint cartilage by supporting and enhancing chondrocyte synthesis:

- Supporting or enhancing the synthesis of synovial fluid, which is required to lubricate the joint.

- Inhibiting free radical enzymes and autoimmune processes that degrade joint cartilage.

- Removing blockages in blood vessels leading to the joint.

A glucosamine deficiency caused by faulty diet, trauma, and aging contributes to the development of osteoarthritis. European studies have shown that the oral administration of glucosamine produced major reductions in joint pain, joint tenderness, and swelling. Improvements in joint function and overall physical performance were noted, compared with placebo and/or ibuprofen. While ibuprofen worked more rapidly than glucosamine in relieving pain, glucosamine had more long-lasting results because it became incorporated into the joint cartilage matrix, resulting in healthier cartilage and less damage to the joints. However, although glucosamine is highly promising, recent research shows that it may not be entirely free of side effects that might affect the muscles, nervous system, or kidneys.

Nutritional Supplements

Welcome to the often-bewildering world of neutraceuticals, nonprescription nutritional supplements that are purported to be helpful in alleviating various illnesses—in this case, arthritis. I say "bewildering" because many of these remedies have been popularized through hearsay, folk wisdom, or anecdotal evidence. There may be some truth to the contention that they work, but I can't vouch for them with any certainty. The most reliable evidence is obtained through the scientific "gold standard" of clinical studies, which are often notably absent with neutraceuticals. I am listing these remedies here for the sake of completeness. Since they are reputed to be helpful, and do not appear to do harm, they may be worth trying.

It is important to recognize that the kind of people who are motivated enough to start taking nutritional supplements usually do not begin taking these supplements in a vacuum. Taking nutritional supplements is often accompanied by other lifestyle changes, such as the elimination of unhealthful foods from the diet, the incorporation of regular exercise into the schedule, and the adoption of stress-reduction techniques.

- **MSM (Methyl-Sulfonyl-Methane).** MSM is a natural form of sulfur found in many fresh foods, including most fresh fruits and vegetables, milk, and some grains. Even though MSM is present in fresh foods, it is easily destroyed in cooking, storing, and processing, and sufficient MSM levels may not be present to provide significant biological sulfur. MSM should be used for cartilage repair and joint lubrication in OA only.

- **Ginger.** Raw, candied, or cooked ginger seems to help people with OA. Ginger supplements are also available at health food stores.

- **Vitamins and Minerals.** Multivitamin and mineral supplements, including vitamins C, E, the B group (especially B_6, B_{12}, and B_3), A, and D, may be helpful. Mineral supplements should include magnesium, calcium, zinc, and iron.

- **Piasclédine.** Piasclédine, a drug used in parts of Europe, is an extract from soybean and avocado. A limited number of reliable studies have shown that it brought about some improvement in mild to moderate arthritis symptoms after a few months. However, it had less impact on patients with severe symptoms.

Rub-On Balms

Some topical ointments offer relief for arthritis without systemic side effects, including Ben Gay, Aspercreme, Myoflex, Mineral Ice, Icy Hot, Absorbine Jr., Mentholatum, Heet, Zeel, and Traumeel. They cause the blood vessels to expand and the area to feel warm, bringing relief. Usually, however, the relief is short-lived and quite local. The very advantage of a topical ointment—that it doesn't enter the system—is also its disadvantage, because its beneficial effects don't go beyond the confines of the immediate area.

Heat and Cold

Moist heat (such as a warm bath or shower) or dry heat (such as a heating pad) placed on the painful area of the joint for about fifteen minutes may relieve the pain. An ice pack (or a bag of frozen veg-etables) wrapped in a towel and placed on the sore area for about fifteen minutes may help to reduce swelling and stop the pain. (Do not use cold packs if you have poor circulation.)

Additional Treatments for Arthritis

Acupuncture. In acupuncture, a medical approach that originated in China, thin needles are inserted at specific points in the body. The National Institutes of Health (NIH) has endorsed the use of acupuncture for pain relief. Scientists think that application of the needles at appropriate points may stimulate the release of natural, pain-relieving chemicals produced by the brain or the nervous sys-tem. The United States now has an accreditation procedure for acupuncturists. Make sure that the one you consult has proper qualifications. It would be helpful if he or she also has experience dealing with arthritis and other inflammatory conditions.

Massage. Lightly stroking and/or kneading a painful muscle may increase blood flow and bring warmth to an affected area. How-ever, because arthritis-stressed joints are very sensitive, you need to find a massage therapist with experience in dealing with arthrit-ic patients. An inexperienced masseur or masseuse might cause further injury to the joint.

Using a splint or a brace. Wearing a splint or brace to allow joints to rest and/or protect them from injury can be helpful.

Other treatments for arthritis include hydrotherapy, heat mas-sage, cold massage, ultrasound (deep heat), hot wax (heat thera-py), traction, transcutaneous electrical nerve stimulation (TENS), biofeedback, psychological counseling, and meditation. Each of these approaches offers some hope and may represent a partial solution to the arthritis problem.

GREEN-LIPPED MUSSEL LIPID OIL

It is the contention of this book that over and above healthful lifestyle changes, the lipid oil extract of the green-lipped mussel is the most effective and also the safest nutraceutical supplement for arthritis. It's also more effective and safer than pharmaceutical medications. Although OA and RA are caused by different disease processes, they have much in common. Both respond well to fish oils in general and the lipid oil in particular. Remember that the lipid oil affects two different pathways—LOX and COX—responsible for inflammation, and it manages to do this without causing any of the adverse effects associated with existing anti-arthritis medications, such as NSAIDs. Let's take a closer look at some of the studies that support the beneficial impact of the green-lipped mussel lipid oil extract on arthritis.

- After more than twenty years of research, clinical trials have shown this lipid oil extract to be more effective in reducing arthritic pain and inflammation than other remedies. Additional clinical trials have demonstrated that this lipid oil can outperform proprietary pharmaceutical NSAIDs as well as remedies such as the traditional fish and plant oils containing omega-3 and omega-6 fatty acids.

- French researchers conducted a six-month randomized study of the effects of stabilized mussel powder on OA of the knee. Of 53 patients, 27 received stabilized mussel powder every day and 26 received a placebo. Patients' symptoms were measured at the beginning and end of the study, and at one-month intervals during the study. For the first five months, neither group of patients showed any change in symptoms. Then, toward the end of the study, patients with mild to moderate forms of OA experienced symptom relief. Those with more serious symptoms experienced no change, even after six months. The results, though modest, did hold promise because none of those taking the placebo improved at all.

- In 2000, Dr. Michael Whitehouse of the University of Queensland, Australia, compared Celebrex and Vioxx, two COX-2 inhibitors, with the lipid oil extract from green-lipped mussels and also with Anaprox, an NSAID (naproxen) in clinical use since 1972, in laboratory rats. At a dosage rate of 15 mg/kg of body weight/day, Celebrex and the lipid oil protected against experimentally induced arthritic inflammation in the rats about equally (78% reduction in inflammation). Vioxx did not reduce inflammation until the dosage was raised significantly, and then it reduced inflammation only minimally. Anaprox appeared to score well, reducing inflammation by over 80%. However, it also created the largest number of gastric side effects. The other agents did not produce any gastric disturbance. Dr. Whitehouse concluded that the green-lipped mussel oil extract was as effective as Celebrex and had no adverse side effects.

• A stabilized freeze-dried powder preparation of whole green-lipped mussels from New Zealand given orally to rats showed some modest anti-inflammatory activity. More important, it strikingly reduced the incidence of stomach ulcers in rats that were taking other NSAIDs, such as aspirin and indomethacin. This implies that not only is this lipid oil extract free of negative side effects, but that it may actually protect against side effects induced by other medications.

• Studies carried out by Dr. Whitehouse comparing the effectiveness of green-lipped mussel oil extract with that of the prescription drug indomethacin showed that, with a dosage of 5 mg/kg of body weight, the oil extract was 97% effective in reducing swelling. In comparison, indomethacin, which is toxic at this dosage, was only 83% effective.

• Dr. Whitehouse and his colleagues recently compared the lipid oil to forty over-the-counter remedies, including three NSAIDs, and found it to be superior to all of them.

• In 1980, research groups from the Homeopathic Hospital and the Department of Surgery, Victoria Infirmary, Glasgow, Scotland, reported on a randomized study involving 66 outpatients, 28 with RA and 38 with OA. All had failed to respond to conventional treatments and had been scheduled for surgery to improve their joint conditions. These patients were randomly divided into two groups. For three months, group one received the powdered mussel (unstabilized) extract and group two received a placebo (dried fish-meal powder). Evaluations were done on day ninety. Then all patients were given the powdered mussel extract for three additional months. At the end of that period, results showed that 68% of RA and 39% of OA patients experienced improvement. No side effects were attributed to the mussel powder. Again, the authors concluded that the powdered mussel extract is an effective supplement or possible alternative to other therapies in the treatment of both RA and OA. It reduced the amount of pain and stiffness, improved the patients' ability to cope with life, and apparently enhanced general health.

• Drs. Robin Gibson and Sheila Gibson continued to explore the effectiveness of the New Zealand green-lipped mussel oil extract. When the lipid oil became available, they began a study comparing mussel powder (Seatone) to the oil. There were 60 patients in the study comparing Seatone powder with the lipid oil—30 with RA and 30 with OA. The patients in each category were randomly assigned to receive either the lipid oil or the stabilized powdered extract. All previous therapy was left unaltered and no other treatment was given throughout the six months of the trial.

The double-blind section of the trial was continued for three months, after which all patients were given the lipid oil for a further three months. After the final three months, the patients were assessed. The results were impressive: 76% of RA and 70% of OA patients benefited. Again the investigators concluded that the green-lipped mussel oil extract is effective in reducing pain, swelling, and stiffness, and in improving function.

• In Denmark—a cold, damp climate—about 10% of the population age twenty-four to seventy-four has acute OA symptoms. Researchers conducted a pilot study of the effects of green-lipped mussel oil on OA. Thirteen patients with long-standing OA in one or both knees and/or hips were included. Of the 13 patients, 12 reported less pain at the first evaluation three to four weeks after commencement of the treatment. This result was maintained at the second evaluation. As expected, the pain relief was accompanied by a considerable improvement in functional ability. Only one patient who completed the trial reported no significant functional improvement. The scientists concluded that the lipid oil extract seemed to be an exceedingly potent drug against pain from OA.

- A double-blind study conducted at the Queen Mary Hospital of the University of Hong Kong compared the effects of green-lipped mussel oil vs. placebo on the signs and symptoms and quality of life in patients with osteoarthritis of the knee. Eighty patients with knee OA were randomized to receive either the lipid oil or placebo for six months. All were allowed paraceta-mol/acetaminophen (Tylenol) rescue treatment to control pain during the study and were reviewed regularly for assessment of arthritis and safety evaluation. Assessment of each patient's OA included the use of a standard 100 mm visual analog scale (VAS) to allow the patient to "quantify" his/her pain, patient's and physician's global assessment of OA, a validated Chinese version of a specific knee score (COKS), a validated Chinese version of a core addressing the impact of arthritis (CAIMS2-SF), and two laboratory common tests—erythrocyte sedimentation rate (ESR) and C-reactive protein (CRP), both considered as valid markers of active inflammation.

  Improvement in almost all of the arthritis assessment variables was observed in both groups of patients, emphasizing the need for placebo-controlled studies; the placebo effect may be important and may lead to false, optimistic conclusions. However, there was a significantly greater improvement in the perception of pain (VAS) and patient's global assessment of OA in those who took the mussel lipid oil when compared to those who had received the placebo; this significant difference persisted even after adjusting for the amount of paracetamol/acetaminophen (Tylenol) consumed to control the pain. This was observed from week four, confirming the slow effect of the lipid oil. Patients who took the lipid oil but not placebo also had improved scores in the CAIMS2-SF physical and psychological domains from week four, meaning an improved quality of life. The mussel oil extract was safe and well tolerated by all patients.

- Dr. Se-Haeng Cho of Yonsei Medical Clinic, in Seoul, Korea, organized a multicenter two-month clinical trial with a total of eight specialized clinics. Sixty patients with symptomatic, painful OA of the knee and hip were included to receive mussel lipid oil at a dose of two capsules twice daily. The physicians analyzed the following: pain according to VAS; an international index designed by Dr. Michel Lequesne (Lequesne index); global assessment by the patient and by the physician; and adverse effects. The treatment with the lipid oil led to significant improvement of the signs and symptoms of OA as determined by all efficacy measurements. After the four- and eight-week treatment periods, 53% and 80%, respectively, of patients experienced significant pain relief and improvement of joint function. There were no reported adverse effects attributable to the green-lipped mussel oil.

- In Germany, a group of physicians studied the efficacy and tolerability of a combination of the green-lipped mussel lipid oil and high concentrations of the fish oils EPA and DHA in patients with rheumatoid arthritis (RA). This twelve-week study was conducted on 50 adults, both men and women. A total of 34 patients required drug therapy before and during the study. But by the end of the study, 21 (62%) were able to reduce their dosage and, more importantly, 13 were able to terminate all medications. At week twelve, 38% were symptom free, and the number of patients complaining of severe pain decreased significantly from 60% (at the beginning of the study) to 25% at the completion of the trial. That special combination of the lipid extract of the green-lipped mussels and selected omega-3 fatty acids was very well tolerated, with just one episode of transient mild nausea.

THE LIPID OIL AND OTHER RHEUMATOLOGICAL CONDITIONS

A number of other conditions mimic or include the inflammatory effects of RA and OA. Two that we know have responded to treatment by the lipid oil extract are gout and ankylosing spondylitis.

Gout

Gout, which has been called the "disease of kings and the king of diseases," has been known, defined, and studied since the days of the ancient Greek physician Hippocrates. Formerly a leading cause of painful and disabling chronic arthritis, gout has been all but conquered by effective treatments. Unfortunately, this information has been slow to spread to physicians and patients.

Gout, which affects an estimated 840 out of every 100,000 people, is a type of arthritis caused by an excess of uric acid in the body. People who have gout either produce too much uric acid or they cannot properly eliminate it from their bodies. While the mussel lipid oil is very helpful in treating gout and has been approved as a treatment for gout by the Australian government, it will be far more effective if it is used in conjunction with prescription medication. Always check with your health care provider before combining any medications.

Ankylosing Spondylitis

Ankylosing spondylitis is an inflammatory condition that affects the spine by fusing the vertebrae together. It is very serious and can even be life-threatening. Current anti-inflammatory drugs have only limited effectiveness and have serious side effects. While controlled studies have been unconvincing to date, anecdotal evidence suggests that the mussel lipid oil may be effective in reducing inflammatory symptoms of this devastating disease. One patient, herself a physician, was unable to use the standard pharmaceutical medication (indomethacin) because of serious side effects. She began taking the mussel lipid oil and now reports being symptom-free. Further studies are needed to replicate this extraordinary case history.

4

Cardiovascular Disease

- *Every 29 seconds, an American suffers a heart attack. And every minute, an American dies from a heart attack.*

- *Every 53 seconds, an American has a stroke. And every 3.3 minutes, an American dies from a stroke.*

- *One in five Americans has some form of cardiovascular illness, resulting in such life-threatening conditions as heart disease and strokes.*

- *Every year, about 600,000 Americans suffer strokes, and an estimated 22% of the nearly 4.5 million stroke survivors are permanently disabled.*

- *Close to one in two women dies from cardiovascular disease.*

- *Eliminating all forms of cardiovascular disease would raise life expectancy in the United States by almost seven years.*

- *Cardiovascular disease costs the U.S. an estimated $327 billion per year. Heart disease is the leading cause of disability in the U.S. labor force, accounting for 19% of Social Security disability payments.*

The most disturbing aspect of these statistics is that they are not necessary! Cardiovascular disease is preventable. It is brought on by many of the unhealthy lifestyle factors we discussed in Chapter 3 in connection with joint disorders, including a diet too rich in trans-fatty acids, excessive consumption of omega-6 fatty acids unbalanced by the omega-3 group, and a sedentary and high-stress lifestyle.

All of these factors overtax the cardiovascular system. Being too oil rich in omega-6 fatty acids inflames the inner lining of the arteries, and opens the gates to the formation of plaques rich in cholesterol. A high intake of trans-fatty acids makes the blood thicker and more "gluey" in consistency. The blood moves slowly through the vessels, rather than efficiently, and it is more likely to get "gummed up" along the way, leading to dangerous blood clots. The extra fat builds a lining of plaque along the walls of the blood vessels, which makes them less elastic and also narrower, so the blood has additional trouble passing through. The condition of plaque buildup along artery walls is called atherosclerosis and is largely responsible for cardiovascular disease—especially stroke and heart attack—in Western countries.

THE BENEFITS OF OMEGA-3 FISH OILS

Incorporating more omega-3 fatty acids into the diet reduces the negative impact of the omega-6 and the trans-fatty acids. Scientists are not entirely sure if this apparent protection is directly related to the capacity of omega-3 fatty acids to dilute viscous blood and prevent atherosclerosis or whether it is mediated through some other means not directly related to fat metabolism. Inflammation and atherosclerosis share similar biochemical mechanisms, at least in their early phases. This commonality has given rise to some fruitful avenues of research into the mechanism of atherosclerosis and its prevention.

It appears that the omega-3 polyunsaturated fatty acids (PUFAs) modify the lipid (fat) content in the blood. They increase concentrations of high-density lipoprotein (HDL-2), the "good" cholesterol, and also increase the levels of "good" triglyceride-rich concentration of lipoproteins (proteins bonded to fats), but they keep levels of undesirable cholesterol and triglycerides down. The excessive amount of blood fat often present after a heavy meal can be reduced by omega-3 PUFAs, although it may sound strange to use a fat to combat another fat.

Additional benefits of omega-3 fish oils include improvements in the walls of the arteries: the endothelium (the lining along the blood-vessel walls) functions more effectively and the arteries become more elastic. This flexibility is important because it allows blood to flow more rapidly and efficiently. How does fish oil promote elasticity? By preventing the formation and accumulation of atherosclerotic plaque. This, in turn, is accomplished by inhibiting the growth of the cells that form the plaque.

Combating atherosclerosis is just one of many functions performed by marine-based omega-3 fats. Fish oils reduce the risk of thrombosis. Eicosapentaenoic acid (EPA), an anti-inflammatory product of the omega-3 group, prevents thrombosis by inhibiting the synthesis of thromboxane A_2, the prostaglandin that causes blood clotting and vascular constriction.

Even if fish oil made no other contribution to human health beyond reducing the incidence of thrombosis, we'd be dealing with an invaluable substance. But fish oil also inhibits the synthesis of low-density lipoprotein (LDL), the "bad" cholesterol. It even has a mild blood pressure–lowering effect in both normal and mildly hypertensive individuals.

The beneficial actions of fish oils are not confined to the blood vessels. The EPA and DHA in fish oils have been shown to correct ventricular fibrillation in the heart. The ventricles are two of the heart's four chambers that, under normal circumstances, beat in a rhythmic and methodical way. Ventricular fibrillation is a very rapid, uncoordinated series of fluttering contractions of the heart's ventricles. The heartbeat and pulse beat are no longer functioning in synchrony, a dangerous situation that can lead to heart failure.

GREEN-LIPPED MUSSEL OIL AS PART OF A HEART-FRIENDLY LIFESTYLE

Most of studies that show EPA and DHA to be effective in addressing cardiovascular disease were carried out using an array of fish oils other than this mussel lipid oil extract, but their findings also apply to the efficacy of the extracted oil of green-lipped mussels. As we saw in Chapter 2, very small quantities of the lipid oil are often more potent than very large quantities of fish oil. It's fair to say that any study confirming the effectiveness of fish oil can be applied to this lipid oil extract. It can even be assumed that the mussel oil will heighten and magnify the effect of the fish oil being studied, since it is much more concentrated and contains so many different types of PUFAs.

Although this is a fair assumption, studies have been performed to investigate whether or not this lipid oil extract is actually more effective than other fish oils. For example, one researcher compared the effectiveness of two marine oils—Fishaphos (a commercial fish oil sold in Australia) and the mussel lipid oil extract. The lipid oil slightly lowered both total and LDL cholesterol and reduced blood pressure, while the other fish oil increased both.

The lipid oil of the green-lipped mussels is not a panacea and will not fully offset the negative impact of a destructive lifestyle. Rather, it should be incorporated into an overall program to enhance your cardiovascular system, which includes the dietary changes we discussed in the chapter on arthritis. While they were recommended in connection with preserving the health of your joints, they will also preserve the health of your heart.

Exercise is also crucial. It keeps the blood vessels toned and the circulation brisk, so that oxygen is transported to your organs more efficiently. It also helps to keep blood fat levels low.

Stress does great damage to the heart. The mechanism through which this happens is called the "fight-or-flight response." This phrase refers to an ancient, primeval defense mechanism programmed into our body, a mechanism that kicks in when we feel threatened. It appears to have originated in the bodies of our primitive ancestors, who had to confront physical danger on a regular basis. When they were about to be attacked by some predatory beast, their adrenaline rose. In response, their heartbeat sped up and blood went racing through their bodies, feeding oxygen to muscles and priming them to spring into action—either to fight the beast or to flee from it. Both courses of action required massive physical expenditure and the body responded by pumping out maximum energy.

In today's society, we are rarely attacked by raging beasts (at least not four-legged ones). Our "beasts" are more likely to be unpleasant bosses, uncooperative teenagers, or unpaid bills. But our primitive defense system doesn't know that—we react to these "threats" posed by our civilized society with all the same physiological ammunition that we would apply to a jungle beast. Our heartbeat speeds up and our palms start to sweat. We want to slug someone—or run away as fast as we can. Because we live in such a stressful world, we are subjected to these "fight-or-flight" triggers many times a day. The strain this puts on the heart and circulatory system is enormous.

So stress-reduction techniques will help not only your joints, but also your heart. Harvard cardiologist Herbert Benson suggested meditation in his book *The Relaxation Response.* He said that the way to counterbalance the fight-or-flight response is to create a "relaxation response." Counseling might also be a helpful way to look at the sources of stress in your life and examine how you might change them or at least see them in a different light if they cannot be changed.

GREEN-LIPPED MUSSEL OIL IS NOT A BLOOD THINNER

"You can't be too rich or too thin," the saying goes. Where blood is concerned, that's not entirely true. Although we don't want blood to be thick and gluey, we also don't want it to be too thin. It needs a certain amount of clotting factor, or you will bleed too easily; and when you bleed, you won't be able to stop quickly enough. Studies have shown that fish oils increased the risk of excessive bleeding while the green-lipped mussel lipid oil extract had no effect on clotting, which means that it is safe even when taken together with aspirin or other blood-thinning medications, such as Coumadin (warfarin).

Why is this lipid extract effective without some of the more problematic side effects associated with aspirin, Coumadin, and even other fish oils? Perhaps it's because the mussel oil does not affect a particular group of clotting factors, such as prothrombin, that are made in the liver. Its action appears to work on the level of thromboxane, another clotting factor, which is manufactured via the COX-2 pathway. Because this lipid oil does not disturb some of the major clotting factors that originate in the liver but still works against other clotting factors, it protects and maintains the ability of the blood to clot appropriately when injury is sustained.

5

Asthma and Allergies

Dimitri, 35, is a respiratory therapist who suffered from exercise-induced asthma, especially in cold weather. If he ran or climbed stairs, for example, he began to cough and wheeze. His symptoms did not clear up until he rested and took his "rescue" remedy—one to three puffs of the bronchodilator albuterol. Dimitri also experienced episodes of wheezing that woke him up during the night. His peak expiratory flow—a standard measure of the ability of an asthmatic person to exhale—was 15% below normal.

Dimitri also suffered from skin problems. These began with atopic dermatitis (infantile eczema), which lasted until age 8; even once the most severe symptoms abated, his skin remained dry and brittle. His nose was always congested, and he suffered from night thirst and loud snoring. Severe allergies run in his family—his mother and sister both suffer from asthma.

Eight months after starting treatment with the green-lipped mussel oil extract, Dimitri experienced notable improvements. He was able to reduce his use of "rescue" inhalers from two canisters to one canister of medication per month. He has also stopped snoring, a sign of less night-time obstruction of the airways. Best of all, his peak expiratory flow became normal.

Millions of people worldwide suffer from asthma, which is one of the most common chronic diseases. Asthma is often allergic in nature and is one of several manifestations of allergy, which is a typical profile of asthmatic individuals. Although asthma affects people of all ages, its incidence is increasing at an alarming rate in children. It occurs in all countries regardless of the level of economic development, but appears to be slightly more common in poor and minority populations than among affluent Caucasians.

In the United States, asthma affects an estimated 17 million Americans—more than 6% of the population—including nearly 5 million children. The disease is responsible for more than 14 million outpatient visits to health care professionals, nearly half a million hospitalizations, more than 1 million emergency room visits, and more than 5,000 deaths annually. Costs associated with asthma are staggering—approximately $6.2 billion per year, including both direct medical costs ($3.6 billion) and indirect costs resulting from reduced productivity, such as missed days at work or school ($2.6 billion). These grim circumstances persist despite our progress in understanding asthma and its underlying inflammatory component.

WHAT IS ASTHMA?

Asthma is a chronic disorder of the airways within the lungs and/or leading to the lungs. As these airways become inflamed, they thicken and become less elastic and also narrower. The result is that airflow to the lungs is limited. Over time, as the asthma worsens, the situation becomes exacerbated. These exacerbations can be severe and even result in death unless effective treatment is initiated.

Asthma has recently been redefined by the National Heart, Lung, and Blood Institute (NHLBI) as "a chronic inflammatory disorder of the airways in which many cells and cellular elements play a role, in particular, mast cells, eosinophils, T-lymphocytes, neutrophils, and epithelial cells." By now, some of these names should be familiar to you. For example, you encountered mast cells in our discussion of joints. They are cells within the cartilage that release pro-inflammatory chemicals. Epithelial cells reside along the lining of internal body cavities, such as the airways leading to the lungs. Eosinophils are usually present when some allergic process is taking place in the body.

74

Although asthma involves inflammation of the airways leading to the lungs, it also involves chronic inflammation within the lungs themselves. When that happens, the person develops respiratory symptoms, such as over-reactivity of the airways and airflow limitation. The bronchi narrow and become constricted, the airway walls swell and change shape (this is called "remodeling"), and the airways become blocked by mucus plugs.

The concept of asthma as an inflammatory disorder is a relatively recent one. Prior to the 1980s, asthma was considered to result primarily from contraction of the smooth muscles in the airways, and asthma treatment consisted primarily of bronchodilators (medications that expand the bronchi). Although asthma continues to increase in prevalence, scientists have been moving ahead with new understanding and treatment. It is hoped that these advances will eventually catch up with the galloping rise of the disease and we will see significant decreases in its incidence and severity.

Inflammation is now known to be a key element in the development of asthma, suggesting numerous potential mechanisms by which asthma may be controlled. For example, knowledge of the importance of leukotrienes has led to the recent development of antileukotriene agents, the first new class of drugs for the treatment of asthma in twenty-five years. The hope is that new therapies to deal with inflammation by targeting specific molecules involved in asthma will help patients and health care providers better manage this disease.

ASTHMA AND INFLAMMATION

In susceptible individuals, inflammation causes recurrent episodes of wheezing, breathlessness, chest tightness, and cough, particularly at night and/or in the early morning. These symptoms are usually associated with widespread but variable airflow limitation that is at least partly reversible, either spontaneously or with treatment. The inflammation also causes an associated increase in airway responsiveness to a variety of stimuli.

Asthma inflammation is mediated through several different types of inflammatory cells. Among the major offenders are those produced by the two inflammatory pathways, cyclo-oxygenase (COX) and lipoxygenase (LOX). The suffix "-ase" at the end of both words means that the offending agents are enzymes. Enzymes are proteins that help break down other substances to form new substances. In the case of asthma, there is a series of "breakdown" cells resulting from both pathways.

When invaders enter our body, our body releases "fighter" cells to "vanquish" the invaders. These cells include eosinophils and monocytes, which are formed in the bone marrow. They enter the blood and migrate to the affected tissue in the body—in this case, the lungs. There, the monocytes differentiate into macrophages, which rove about devouring unwelcome organisms. Additional processes that take place during inflammation are the buildup of blood platelets in contact with the affected area, the involvement of chemicals released by mast cells, and the shedding of cells along the epithelium or lining.

Let's increase the magnification on our microscopes and look more closely at the eosinophils. They contain a variety of pre-formed mediators and, through a series of chemical reactions, they form leukotrienes in their membranes—the chemicals we've already encountered in the inflammatory process in the joints.

Asthma usually doesn't strike in a vacuum—typically, it is triggered by an allergic reaction. The food or environmental particle that triggers this reaction is called an allergen. Allergic patients manufacture specific antibodies (IgE) against these allergens. These Y-shaped antibodies anchor into a membrane receptor of mast cells, located in the bronchi, nose or skin. When the allergic patient, who is loaded with IgE attached to mast cells, re-encounters the pollen or dust to which he is allergic, the contact between the IgE and the allergen will trigger the release of powerful inflammatory mediators: histamine, leukotrienes, and more. These toxic, pro-inflammatory substances will dilate the blood vessels; the capillaries will leak, generating swelling; the nerve ending will be tickled, with a resulting intolerable itch; the skin or the nose will turn red; the asthmatic will choke due to mucus plugging the wind pipes. And the body releases eosinophils to combat the allergens! These eosinophils, in turn, release substances that trigger mast cells to release histamine and leukotrienes. When you go to the pharmacy to buy an antihistamine to combat some allergic reaction, you're buying a drug that fights histamine. Histamine and leukotrienes have the same impact on the airways leading to the lungs—they cause these airways, which are made of smooth muscle, to contract.

Taking antihistamines might help you stop sneezing if you're allergic to cats and your neighbor just presented you with a kitten. It might help your rash if you have come in contact with poison ivy—which is, ultimately, an allergic reaction to the oils exuded by the poison ivy leaves. By combating histamine, these medications can be crucial and even lifesaving. However, they are not sufficient to combat asthma by themselves. Antihistamines will not address the central role that leukotrienes play in the contraction of the smooth airway muscles, which is the consequence of an inflammatory response. Leukotrienes are 100 to 1,000 times more broncho-constricting than histamine. Their effect is also far more prolonged. Leukotrienes don't just lead to the tightening of the bronchial passages. They also stimulate mucus production. They make the tiny blood vessels more permeable, allowing allergens to enter them, and they cause the eosinophils to migrate to new areas, where the inflammatory process starts all over again. This is how they're responsible for the worsening of asthmatic symptoms.

You may be able to guess which acid is responsible for leukotriene synthesis: our old friend, arachidonic acid. And by now you also understand how to reduce the amount of arachidonic acid by adopting dietary and other lifestyle changes (covered in Chapter 3). As you'll see, the green-lipped mussel lipid oil extract can also play a role in reducing the inflammation associated with asthma.

Gloria, 16, suffered from serious asthma. She had always been prone to allergies and had experienced her first major attack of food-induced hives as an infant. At 4, she developed asthma, which continued throughout her childhood and adolescence. She needed to use her beta-agonist inhaler many times each day and woke up wheezing at least once every night. When the inhaler was ineffective, her parents assisted her in using a nebulizer, a machine that delivers medicine to the lungs via mist. Even with the home-based nebulizer, she experienced periodic uncontrollable asthma attacks that required trips to the emergency room.

Gloria began taking corticosteroids at age 10. They curtailed the asthma attacks somewhat, but caused yeast infections and weight gain that finally forced her to discontinue use after five years. For much of the time, Gloria was irritable, tense, and volatile. She was constantly tired due to interrupted sleep and also due to the side effects of her medications.

When she began taking the green-lipped mussel oil, Gloria noticed an immediate reduction in her asthma symptoms. Within a matter of days, she stopped waking up during the night. After a week, she needed her inhaler only once a day. Her mood began to improve and her family noticed that she had become much easier to live with. Now, Gloria is thriving and hopes her progress will continue.

CURRENT TREATMENT APPROACHES TO ASTHMA

Recognition of the important role that inflammation plays in asthma has led to increased emphasis on anti-inflammatory agents to treat the disease. Extensive research efforts are seeking to identify the inflammatory mechanisms associated with asthma and to develop new anti-inflammatory treatments. While control of an asthma attack is still a crucial aspect of asthma therapy, greater attention is being paid to prevention and management of the chronic inflammatory aspects of the disease.

Asthma is a complex disease in which episodic attacks are superimposed on a chronic inflammatory condition in the lung. The various drugs prescribed by doctors are aimed at different components of the disease. Let's look at a few of the most widely prescribed medications.

Antihistamines

Histamine is one of the major mediators released from the mast cell in allergic reactions; therefore, preventing its ability to stimulate target organs has become an obvious goal in drug development. Antihistamines are not sufficient to control all aspects of the disease, however, because they do not address the role that leukotrienes play in the vicious cycle of asthma.

Relievers and Controllers

These are two major categories of drugs aimed at providing relief from asthma symptoms as quickly as possible. As we have seen, asthma is not only a spasm; it's an inflammation, a thickening of the tissue inside the airways. A spasm can be relieved very quickly, but inflammation takes much longer to heal. If something is swollen, it may take hours or even days to go down. As the name implies, relievers are designed to bring symptomatic relief: they "despasm" the muscle, so to speak. Bronchodilators dilate or stretch the contracted bronchial muscles. They do not, however, address the full range of symptoms. For example, they are not designed to break up plugs of mucus or to heal inflammation. For those purposes, we have a second category of medication, called the controllers. The two major controllers are the corticosteroids and the antileukotrienes.

Corticosteroids have been the drug of choice for treating chronic severe asthma since 1950. Although the anti-inflammatory role of steroids was not recognized and understood when these powerful medications were first being prescribed, it is now known that treating milder asthma with corticosteroids may also help to reduce bronchial inflammation and control the progression of the disease. However, systemic corticosteroids, albeit potent and effective medications, have potentially debilitating side effects, particularly affecting the kidneys, the bones, and the adrenal glands. Some recent research has linked corticosteroids with thyroid disease, mood swings, yeast infections, and a host of other disturbing conditions. Plus, oral corticosteroids are notorious for causing weight gain.

Inhaled corticosteroids are often used as the primary long-term controller therapy for asthma. Although corticosteroid therapy is believed to work by suppressing airway inflammation, it's still not entirely clear exactly how the mechanics of this process work. One study suggested that perhaps corticosteroids reduced the number of inflammatory eosinophils that migrate to the affected tissues. Another theory suggests that corticosteroids may control the production of inflammatory mediators.

Other long-term control therapies are mast cell stabilizers, which inhibit the release of inflammatory mediators by mast cells. They include DSCG/cromolyn and nedocromil—medications called cromones—that are considered safer than corticosteroids because they have a more favorable side-effect profile. However, they are also less effective in long-term control. Their anti-inflammatory action is only mild, although they are somewhat more versatile than corticosteroids because they inhibit early-phase responses to allergens as well as chronic allergic-inflammatory reactions.

Adrenaline (also called epinephrine) has been used to relieve asthma symptoms for about ninety years. It is a very powerful bronchodilator that works by activating the adrenergic receptors. When these receptors in the airways are activated, they are primed and ready to receive the adrenaline, which can then start to work within the lungs. Short-acting, more specific beta-2 agonists are the most powerful bronchodilators available: they include albuterol (Ventolin, Proventil), terbutaline, pirbuterol, bitolterol, and levalbuterol. Bronchodilators are delivered by inhalation to ensure rapid onset of action and to minimize adverse effects. They are the therapy of choice for relieving acute symptoms and preventing exercise-induced bronchospasm.

Adrenaline also inhibits mast cell mediator secretion and constricts the peripheral blood vessels, causing the heart to pump faster. (In fact, it is the chemical responsible for the "rush" involved in the fight-or-flight response.) However, these are not always desirable effects. Adrenaline places a great strain on the cardiovascular system. People who take the medication report feeling jittery and tense, and many experience palpitations. The consensus at present is that most beta-2 agonists are acceptable as occasional "rescue" remedies but are not suitable for long-term use.

Methylxanthines (extracts from tea and coffee) have been used for almost 700 years to treat bronchial asthma. Today, the predominant methylxanthine in clinical use is theophylline. Its precise mechanism as an anti-asthma drug is somewhat obscure. The major disadvantage with theophylline is that it only works in large doses, but too much theophylline could be toxic. Theophylline also has many undesirable side effects, such as excessively rapid heartbeat, high blood pressure, vomiting, seizures, and even death.

The use of cyclo-oxygenase (COX) inhibitors, such as indomethacin or flurbiprofen, inhibits the production of an important bronchoconstrictor called PGD_2, which is made in the mast cells. While these medications have some beneficial effects during an acute asthma attack induced by allergens, they appear to have little benefit in other forms of chronic asthma. Furthermore, these drugs may precipitate so-called aspirin-induced asthma in a small percentage of patients.

We see that most of the currently available medications contain several major problems. Relievers don't address the root cause of the problem. Controllers bring only limited relief and many are associated with side effects that can range from moderate to severe.

ANTILEUKOTRIENES

The most promising of all currently available asthma medications are the antileukotrienes. I am paying special attention to this class of medication because it appears to have the most long-term effectiveness with the fewest negative effects, and because it is closest in purpose and concept to the green-lipped mussel lipid oil extract.

With the realization that inflammation is a key piece in the asthma puzzle, extensive research efforts have gone into identifying the associated inflammatory mechanisms and developing new anti-inflammatory treatments. Through studies of the mechanism of leukotrienes, the first new class of drugs for the treatment of asthma in twenty-five years—the antileukotrienes—was developed. Antileukotriene agents have made asthma compliance much easier. Patients can take them by mouth rather than by inhaler or injection, and they are relatively free of side effects. They're no-fuss-no-muss medications, and highly effective as well.

Antileukotriene agents fall into two general categories: leukotriene synthesis inhibitors (LTSIs) and leukotriene receptor antagonists (LTRAs). LTSIs act at various locations on the leukotriene synthetic pathway, while LTRAs antagonize leukotriene binding at the leukotriene receptors located in the tissues. In other words,

LTSIs prevent leukotrienes from being formed in the first place; and if leukotrienes are present, LTRAs prevent them from attaching to the tissues and continuing the inflammatory process.

Although leukotrienes are partially responsible for causing the smooth muscles of the bronchi to contract, for the formation of mucus, and for the increased permeability of the blood vessels, their primary role is causing inflammation. Studies have shown antileukotrienes to be effective in reducing the number of leukotrienes and inhibiting the effects of those present, even in the presence of allergens that play a role in stimulating leukotriene production.

GREEN-LIPPED MUSSEL LIPID OIL VERSUS ANTILEUKOTRIENES

In previous chapters, we saw that the mussel lipid oil acts on the LOX and COX pathways to inhibit all sorts of inflammatory culprits, including leukotrienes. So, it stands to reason that it should be an effective anti-asthmatic agent.

Let's start by reviewing the research concerning the mussel lipid oil extract's effectiveness in healing other inflammatory processes. Drs. Ian Shiels and Michael Whitehouse compared green-lipped mussel oil extract to two major antileukotrienes, zafirlukast and montelukast, to see which agent was more effective in relieving arthritis symptoms in laboratory rats. They concluded that both antileukotriene drugs were less effective than the mussel lipid oil. Zafirlukast inhibited swelling by 33% percent and montelukast inhibited it by 71%, but the lipid oil inhibited the swelling by an astounding 96%. These findings are impressive indeed. The green-lipped mussel oil was also shown to be more effective than other oils, both plant and marine based.

What does all this have to do with asthma? A great deal, because like arthritis, asthma is an inflammatory process—leukotrienes play a crucial role in asthma as well as in arthritis. The mussel lipid oil extract does not confine its activity only to the leukotrienes present in joints and responsible for swelling and pain in your knuckles or knees. It also affects the leukotrienes present in your lungs.

A double-blind, placebo-controlled study on asthma was conducted under the guidance of Professor Peter J. Barnes of London, England, at the Pavlov University hospital in Saint Petersburg, Russia, and published in 2002 in the *European Respiratory Journal*. The subjects were 46 patients with atopic asthma (asthma associated with allergies) who had never used steroids but were taking "rescue" medications (beta-2 antagonists, such as Proventil). Green-lipped mussel oil was given to 23 of these patients at a dosage of two capsules twice a day; the other 23 were the control group. The lipid oil yielded great improvement in the clinical symptoms, during the night as well as the daytime, of those patients who took it. There was no similar improvement in the placebo group. The investigators also demonstrated that the bronchial inflammation had been reduced in the lipid oil group. They concluded that beneficial effects of the mussel lipid oil in mildly asthmatic patients were due to its anti-inflammatory effects on airways. The study is currently being extended to moderate and severe asthma patients.

Another striking aspect of this study was that patients who took the lipid oil required their beta-2 antagonist inhalers far less than patients who took the placebo. This is an important finding, because beta-2 antagonists have potentially serious side effects. So, not only is the mussel oil extract free of side effects, it also reduces the need for other medications that do have side effects.

Terje, 38, had suffered from severe allergic rhinitis since age 12. During the spring season, his nose became stuffed, and he would sneeze, rub his eyes, and clear his throat. As the season progressed, he also developed exercise-induced asthma, coughing and wheezing if he attempted to run or walk. The allergy also affected his vision: between March and June, Terje was unable to wear his contact lenses. He experienced some mild relief when he used a blue pollen mask, designed to reduce the amount of pollen he inhaled, but he hated the mask as it was uncomfortable and unsightly.

Terje tried to control his symptoms by using antihistamine therapy, but the medication made him very drowsy—a serious problem, since Terje, a former air force pilot, often must fly a plane for his work as a product manager. Topical corticosteroids caused his nose to start hemorrhaging and allergy shots actually made him collapse. Injected corticosteroids had a devastating impact on his moods, precipitating a psychotic episode.

Terje started taking four capsules of mussel oil extract a day in February, one month before the spring symptoms usually hit. He was amazed by the results—his symptoms were about 80% improved, he could wear his contact lenses, pilot an airplane, and even enjoy a beer without adverse effects such as drowsiness. Best of all, he was able to put the blue pollen mask away. Terje discontinued taking the lipd oil in June, but will continue using it every spring.

ALLERGIES

The mechanisms of allergy are not fully understood, although scientists are beginning to fill in many of the missing pieces of the puzzle. In order to grasp what the current research has to say, it is important to understand what an allergy is and what happens in the body when an allergen invades.

As mentioned, our bodies have an immune system designed to fight invading organisms. Without this immune system, we would fall prey to every illness floating around. In fact, people who are born with diseases that rob them of immunity must live their lives in protective "bubbles" where all foreign organisms can be filtered out. The Acquired Immune Deficiency Syndrome (AIDS) virus robs its victims of their ability to fight off illness. Patients therefore are vulnerable to all sorts of "opportunistic infections," invading organisms that take advantage of the body's inability to fight them off. So, our immune system is a gift and something to be grateful for.

But when the immune system goes awry and begins attacking "friendly" invaders, we have a phenomenon known as allergies. It would be as if the border patrol of a country began taking shots not only at armed and obviously hostile enemy invaders but also at friendly visitors from other countries who arrive with peaceful intentions. So, a person allergic to citrus fruits will react to orange juice as if it were, say, an invading cold virus—by sneezing or sniffling, for example. This might be called a sort of biochemical xenophobia turned inward.

How does this process work? Every offending substance is an antigen, a protein or even a carbohydrate capable of stimulating an immune response. The body responds by releasing antibodies; these are proteins produced by specialized cells after they have been prodded by the presence of the antigen. The antibodies are designed to fight the antigens.

The main class of antibody associated with allergy is immunoglobulin E (IgE). Interestingly, that is also the class of antibody responsible for fighting parasites. If you have a case of intestinal worms, your body will produce a lot of IgE. Is this just coincidence that the same group of antibodies responsible for combating parasites is also responsible for combating allergens? Scientists don't think so—it appears that there actually are tiny living organisms in some apparently inanimate allergens. These microscopic organisms trigger the body's formation of those antibodies that fight parasites. For example, dust—a very common allergen—would appear to be inanimate. What could be alive in a pile of dust? In reality, however, thousands of tiny dust mites live in the dust. Allergic individuals are not reacting to the dust itself but to the mites in the dust.

IgE production is regulated by a series of messengers that we call cytokines (*cyto* means cell and *kine* means move). These cytokines carry the message from the cells that captured the allergen to the cells that produce IgE. The messenger responsible for boosting the production of IgE in allergic individuals is called interleukin-4 (IL-4). "Kill the messenger" may be an inhumane policy when it comes to war and foreign relations, but it's a highly effective policy when it comes to cytokines. It is desirable to slow or destroy IL-4 so that it can't deliver its message to the cells that produce IgE.

IL-4 is not the only messenger on the stage. An allergic reaction is complex—it's not a monologue or one-person show but a group of many actors who come and go. A leukotriene called leukotriene B_4 (LT B_4) is the initial producer and director of the show: it recruits and organizes the actors and gives them their stage commands.

The research of the late Paris-based scientist Dr. Bernard Dugas has shown that the green-lipped mussel lipid oil slows down the activity of IL-4 and reduces LT B_4. This means a much weaker "recruiter" to marshal the actors and no messengers available to transmit the recruiter's instructions. Without a recruiter and a messenger, the IgE-producing cells don't proceed with antibody production and no allergic reaction takes place.

The implications of this research are far-reaching indeed. They suggest that the mussel lipid oil is effective not only in an allergic process such as asthma but also in other allergic reactions, such as skin rashes. Let's have a closer look at the lipid oil extract's effectiveness in helping those who suffer from allergy-induced skin disorders.

DERMATITIS

Dermatitis is an inflammation of the skin that can take many different forms, including swelling, redness, itching, burning, and rashes of different shapes, textures, and sizes. There are two basic forms of dermatitis—atopic (infantile eczema) and contact dermatitis.

Atopic Dermatitis (Infantile Eczema)

Atopic dermatitis (AD) is a chronic, itchy rash that progresses into open, oozing sores. It is caused by an overactive immune system. About 2% of the total population may have atopic dermatitis. It is a disease that favors youth, as the majority of patients are infants and children. The clinical characteristics of atopic dermatitis include the following:

- It affects less than 2% of total population; 80% to 90% affected are five years of age.

- AD is associated with asthma and allergic rhinitis.

- One prominent symptom is hyperirritability of the skin (pruritus).

- Scratching makes it worse and maintains the inflammation.

The clinical manifestations of the disease—both the type of skin lesions as well as their distribution—typically change with age. They can range from acute to mild and may be transient or chronic. AD is not a steady-state disease: patients will cycle from periods of extreme involvement to times when they are symptom-free, and this makes treating the disease frustrating.

The skin of patients with atopic dermatitis is in a constant state of hyperirritability, and itching is the main manifestation that bothers patients. Patients can't seem to stop scratching, which worsens the condition, and a vicious cycle ensues. I call it the chronic itch-scratch cycle and it maintains and worsens the inflammation. While AD affects people of all ages, babies and young children are especially vulnerable, because it is hardest to stop them from scratching. You cannot reason with them verbally, and it is difficult to physically restrain them.

Unlike other allergic reactions, which involve IgE-mediated mechanisms, atopic dermatitis appears to involve other inflammatory substances that infiltrate the skin, including lympho-histiocytic cells. Tiny vesicles form in the outer layer of the skin, the epidermis. There is no obvious involvement of mast cells, nor is there an obvious presence of eosinophils.

Does this mean that there is no IgE or eosinophil involvement in atopic dermatitis whatsoever? Research suggests that there may be some initial role played by eosinophils. Patients with severe generalized atopic dermatitis tend to have very high total serum IgE concentrations. This means that although no IgE is found at the location of the rash, there is a great deal of IgE circulating in their blood. Individuals who suffer from AD tend to produce high concentrations of IgE when they are exposed to common inhalants and even to certain foods.

Sufferers from AD have noticed that when they come in close contact with animals to which they are allergic, they develop a runny nose or asthma. Some develop eczema around the eyes and nose during pollen season. We know that these types of allergic reactions are mediated by the mast cells, through the inflammatory processes we discussed in connection with asthma. So, although some AD patients have normal IgE concentrations, the overlap between those who suffer from AD and those who suffer from other IgE-mediated allergies is too large to be coincidental. It seems likely that the release of leukotrienes during other allergic reactions worsens the AD.

Contact Dermatitis

Allergic contact dermatitis (ACD), a form of delayed hypersensitivity, is a common dermatological problem. If we apply an allergen to the skin of a sensitive patient, an eczematous reaction that is localized to the area of the hypersensitivity response will develop within one to three days. Common contact allergens include:

- Metals such as nickel and cobalt in earring studs, buckles, zippers, fasteners, or jean studs.

- Latex.

- Animal hair and dander.

- Chromium salts in cement, tanned leather, and green textile dyes.

- Paraphenylenediamine (a black dye extracted from coal that is often found in hair dyes and some clothing).

- Medicinal ointments, such as neomycin and synthetic local anesthetics.

- Epoxy resins, fragrances in soaps and toiletries, and creams and ointments containing wood alcohols and parabens.

In many parts of the world, nickel is the most common offending allergen, especially in women with pierced ears. Ingested nickel (occasionally found in water or in poorly maintained cookware) may cause dermatitis in skin that has previously been in contact with nickel. Common allergens differ from continent to continent. In North America, for example, poison oak and poison ivy are common causes of ACD.

Causes of ACD may be immediately apparent or may take considerable sleuthing to define, especially when caused by industrial processes.

GREEN-LIPPED MUSSEL LIPID OIL AND DERMATITIS

Dr. Michael Whitehouse of the University of Queensland, Australia, made two fascinating discoveries regarding the role that mussel lipid oil can play in relieving symptoms of both types of dermatitis. He demonstrated that a topical preparation of lipid extract cured existing dermatitis in animals such as guinea pigs almost as fast as corticosteroids. Even more impressive, he found that if he gave the lipid oil to these animals orally, they did not develop dermatitis when exposed to allergens. The topical preparation requires some fine-tuning if it is to be used effectively for human beings, because it has a foul odor. Meanwhile, mussel lipid oil taken orally can help offset your allergic responses to skin irritants.

ALLERGIC RHINITIS (AR)

Rhinitis is the medical term for those nasty respiratory symptoms you associate with colds—runny nose, nasal congestion, itching, and sneezing. And have you ever wondered whether it's a cold or an allergy? Whether it's some type of upper-respiratory infection, the pollen outside, or the neighbor's cat? Here are a few questions to help you decide:

• Is there a family history of allergies?

• What is your dominant nasal symptom? Is it blockage, sneezes, or runny nose?

• Are the nasal problems isolated or are there more extensive symptoms? For example, what is happening in other parts of the upper airways, such as sinuses or ears? Have you ever suffered from bronchitis, ear infections, or skin problems? A history of bronchitis and ear infections might suggest that a persistent cough or an itchy ear is due to an infection. If you have a rash together with your itchy ears, an allergy seems more likely, especially if you're not prone to ear infections.

• Look around your house. Is it cluttered with lots of "soft" items, such as blankets, carpets, and stuffed toys? Do you have pets?

Do you keep flowering plants in the house? How about out-doors? What types of vegetation grow in your neighborhood? Are you near some type of industrial plant or other source of air pollution?

- What are your occupational and leisure activities and do they aggravate your symptoms?

- Can you find any connection between your symptoms and what you eat or drink?

These questions are designed to give you clues as to what may be going on. Of course, this is not an exhaustive list. If you have any doubt, you should consult your health care practitioner. If infection is ruled out and your AR symptoms don't disappear, you might consult an allergist. These specialists are skilled in ferreting out clues you may not have thought of and testing for reactions to specific substances.

Allergic sensitization seems to occur very early in life when the immune system is immature. Maybe this is the reason why allergic rhinitis is more common in those born in the spring and summer. There is also a higher prevalence of rhinitis in boys than in girls—possibly a genetically determined difference, since IgE levels are higher in boys from birth. Firstborn children are at great-est risk. The relative risk is doubled for children who live in damp houses and/or whose parents smoke. Modern energy-efficient "tight" buildings increase exposure to potential indoor allergens. Environmental pollution is likewise a prime offender.

Recent studies have shown that antileukotrienes are effective against AR, especially when used in conjunction with antihista-mines. People who have tried using the lipid oil of green-lipped mussels together with an antihistamine report that they get far more relief than they did from self-standing antihistamines. While formal scientific studies have not yet been conducted regarding the effectiveness of the mussel lipid oil in alleviating symptoms of AR, the testimonials of those who have tried it are impressive. "My Kleenex bill is way down," said one satisfied user. "I can finally smell the roses!" said another. A third spoke enthusiastically of increased energy and relief from exercise-induced asthma. "I plan to run the New York Marathon!" he announced. One patient reported relief from nighttime congestion and resultant snoring. "Maybe I should look for a wife," he quipped.

CAN YOU BE ALLERGIC TO GREEN-LIPPED MUSSEL LIPID OIL?

The green-lipped mussel lipid oil extract is non-allergenic. To start with, there is no protein and no carbohydrate present in it. Since these are the types of foods that classically induce allergies, the risk of allergy to the lipid oil extract is nonexistent.

I have been contacted by patients who are concerned that they may react poorly to the lipid oil of green-lipped mussels because they are allergic to seafood. I investigated this by contacting the director of the European Research Center on Food Allergies in Nancy, France. Professor Anne-Denise Moneret-Vautrin, the director of the Center, told me that even people who are allergic to mussels will not develop an allergy to mussel oil. She assured me that there is no evidence of IgE-related reactions to any type of mussel oil. Moreover, she has never encountered even a single documented case of such a reaction. The absence of protein and carbohydrate in the oil means that there is no chemical "welcoming committee" for an IgE reaction. So, mussel oil is safe, even if you don't tolerate shellfish.

6

Women's Health Issues

Heather is a 38-year-old laboratory technician. Like all the women in her family, she suffered from "bad veins." She had varicose veins in her legs and uncomfortable hemorrhoids. Due to her vascular problems, high cholesterol, and a pre-diabetic condition, she could not use oral contraceptives, so her gynecologist implanted an intrauterine device (IUD) for birth control.

After that, Heather began experiencing terrible pelvic pain beginning three to four days prior to her period, which worsened during menstruation. She had to take off from work ten days each month. Taking ibuprofen led to a life-threatening uterine hemorrhage and did nothing to alleviate the pain. Other medications she tried caused a host of nasty side effects, including nausea, constipation, mood swings, and dizziness.

Heather started taking four capsules of green-lipped mussel oil daily ten days before her period was expected and discontinued on the last day of her period. For the first time, she experienced no pain, cramps, or excessive bleeding. She followed the same protocol the following month and has continued doing so ever since. She no longer misses any workdays during her menstrual period and reports feeling enormous relief.

Women are different from men. I'm not talking about subtle difference in communicational styles or planetary origins (Mars versus Venus). Women are biochemically different from men, with unique needs emanating from their hormonal cycles. In particular, many women suffer from pain and discomfort during their menstrual periods. The lipid oil of green-lipped mussels has been proven highly effective in addressing dysmenorrhea or painful menstrual periods. Up to 50% of menstruating women suffer from primary dysmenorrhea, at significant economic and social cost. In the United States alone, it has been estimated that 600 million work hours are lost each year due to dysmenorrhea.

How does the green-lipped mussel lipid oil alleviate the pain and discomfort associated with menstruation? First, let's understand what dysmenorrhea is and what it isn't. When we are in pain, we tend to think that something is wrong. We associate physical discomfort with illness. But actually, dysmenorrhea is usually not caused by an illness. Rather, it is associated with increased levels of prostaglandins and/or lipoxygenase (LOX)-produced leukotrienes—both are inflammatory substances, but both are also the triggers of uterine contractions.

As part of its normal physiological function, the uterus contracts rhythmically during menstruation. The force and frequency of these contractions are regulated by hormones—specifically, oxytocin, a hormone synthesized in the pituitary gland. (That's the same hormone that doctors and midwives use to intensify the contractions of women whose labor is progressing too slowly.) Oxytocin stimulates strong uterine contractions and it also acts to increase the local release of eicosanoids.

Elevated concentrations of eicosanoids, such as prostaglandins and leukotrienes, have been identified in women suffering from dysmenorrhea. These mediators increase the force of uterine contractions (more commonly called cramps) and constrict blood vessels. They make pain receptors in the pelvic area exquisitely sensitive to all kinds of physical stimuli or chemicals that induce pain. Under ordinary circumstances, these receptors would be more likely to ignore those stimuli. Now, they're all on red alert. But that's not all they do—the eicosanoids enter the blood circulation and cause general malaise often accompanied by diarrhea, headache, dizziness, and nausea.

Why does the body release these substances during menstruation? Prostaglandins and leukotrienes are physiological mediators of normal uterine contractions and are necessary during menstruation so that the blood will be expelled by the uterus. But when too much production of prostaglandins and leukotrienes takes place, the uterine contractions become too strong and pain develops. While this experience can range from mild discomfort to "please-let-me-lie-down" agony, it is not in and of itself dangerous or pathological.

On the other hand, it's not desirable either. Pain is useful only when it signals the presence of an illness or condition that needs attention. For example, if you break your ankle and experience no pain, you might put weight on the broken bone and worsen the break, rendering your ankle permanently useless. If you come down with strep throat but feel no throat pain, you might never know you have the illness and end up suffering all the potentially dangerous conditions associated with untreated strep. However, here there's no illness being signaled, and therefore no good reason to suffer. What will relieve the pain?

Approximately 80% of women with dysmenorrhea experience symptomatic relief when they are treated with one of the NSAIDs that inhibit the COX enzymes responsible for synthesizing prostaglandins. However, NSAIDs do not give satisfactory relief in approximately 20% of primary dysmenorrhea patients. (Heather is an example of a patient who could not take NSAIDs.) And, of course, NSAIDs have negative side effects. It is common practice to use oral contraceptives to treat these women, but even oral contraceptives are not free of risks.

GREEN-LIPPED MUSSEL LIPID OIL AND DYSMENORRHEA

With the help of the lipid oil extract of green-lipped mussels, it may be possible to reduce the pain you feel during your periods, even without NSAIDs and oral contraceptives. Drs. Ian Shiels and Michael Whitehouse studied uterine contractions in rats. They showed that administering the lipid oil extract of green-lipped mussels to uterine tissue reduces uterine contractions, even when those contractions have been artificially induced by administration of oxytocin.

Why does this oil have this effect on uterine contractions? Studies show that the lipid oil is not a smooth-muscle relaxant, nor does it inhibit any of the chemicals produced by the COX pathway. Rather, it seems to work against the leukotriene receptors in the uterus. If these receptors are blocked, the leukotrienes can't exert their contractive effect on the uterus, and the uterus will consequently be more relaxed.

There is some anecdotal evidence to support the use of the green-lipped mussel lipid oil for dysmenorrhea in humans. Several women suffering from arthritis were taking the lipid oil to alleviate the inflammation in their joints. Some of them also suffered from dysmenorrhea, but did not realize that the oil might alleviate their menstrual discomforts. They were surprised to discover dramatic reductions in their symptoms of dysmenorrhea after they started taking the mussel extract.

The lipid oil of green-lipped mussels is safe for women who are taking oral contraceptives and there is no risk of either excessive clotting or excessive bleeding, even for women who are using intrauterine devices (IUDs).

7

New Directions in Research

We have talked about the extracted lipid oil of the green-lipped mussels as a powerful and effective remedy for arthritis, cardiovascular disease, asthma, and allergies. There are a variety of other situations and conditions in which the lipid oil can be helpful. Scientists studying the lipid oil extract of green-lipped mussels are expanding their investigations into all sorts of new areas. Here are a few of the far-reaching possibilities currently under investigation.

WORKING WITH VACCINES TO STRENGTHEN IMMUNITY

A fascinating double-blind, placebo-controlled study was conducted in 1999—a collaborative project between Russian and Australian scientists—concerning the impact of mussel oil supplementation on the response to influenza vaccination. Subjects were vaccinated with a live, weakened nasal vaccine; then given the lipid oil extract of green-lipped mussels for four weeks. Taken together with the vaccine, the extract greatly strengthened the effectiveness of the vaccine. The findings implied that the lipid oil extract of green-lipped mussels might independently decrease the unwanted inflammatory reaction that we develop when we suffer from the flu (that "achiness" in our joints, for example). And the extract didn't have any negative impact on the normal immune response.

A TREATMENT FOR CANCER?

In 1998 and 1999, Australian scientists applied the lipid oil extract of green-lipped mussels to several lines of cancer cells, and those cells died within twenty-four hours. The cells underwent apoptosis, or programmed cell death. What followed was a great media hubbub, with green-lipped mussel oil extract touted as the upcoming cure for cancer. While there is great hope that this oil might indeed provide a natural alternative for cancer treatment without the side effects of chemotherapy and radiation, that day has not yet arrived.

Research is underway and anecdotal reports have been encouraging. Patients have reported that tumors have shrunk or at least remained unchanged, and tests show that tumor markers have stabilized or decreased. Many patients have experienced relief from pain and a return of appetite. All in all, they report that their quality of life has improved. It remains to be seen, however, whether or not the enthusiastic reports of satisfied patients will be confirmed thorough scientific studies.

INFLAMMATORY BOWEL DISEASE

Inflammatory bowel disease (IBD) is an inflammatory disorder of the digestive tract. It stands to reason that anti-inflammatory agents should alleviate the symptoms of this condition—and that's the rationale behind supplementation with omega-3 polyunsaturated fatty acids (PUFAs), which have anti-inflammatory effects in the body. In fact, the first evidence of the importance of omega-3 PUFAs was derived from epidemiological observations of the low incidence of inflammatory bowel disease in Eskimos.

Crohn's disease is an example of an inflammatory bowel disorder that may be responsive to the lipid oil of green-lipped mussels. The disease is a chronic inflammation of the intestinal tract. Two gastroenterologists in Australia gave the lipid oil extract to two patients who suffered from Crohn's disease—with highly encouraging results. The patients now have normal barium X-rays and physical examination of the rectal area showed no sign of disease. These physicians were so impressed by these promising results that they are planning to conduct a more formal and extensive study.

Researchers in Southern Australia have been using a mouse model of inflammatory bowel disease (inflammatory colitis). They compared the effects of olive oil (control group) with fish oil and the lipid oil extract of green-lipped mussels, using a disease activity index (DAI) to gauge results. The mice fed the mussel lipid oil had a lower DAI: 0 versus 1 for olive oil, and 0 versus 4 for fish oil. Compared with fish oil, the mice given the mussel lipid oil showed a trend for lower overall colitis severity in the distal colon. The green-lipped mussel oil may be potentially useful in ameliorating the symptoms of IBD, as reported anecdotally by the Australian gastroenterologists. This study was recently published in the *Pacific Journal of Clinical Nutrition.*

DIABETES

Diabetes is not a single disease entity but a group of diseases characterized by the body's inability to produce sufficient quantities of insulin. The pancreas doesn't make enough insulin or doesn't make any insulin at all. Sometimes, the pancreas produces enough insulin but the body is unable to utilize it properly.

Insulin is the most important hormone involved in the metabolism of your food. It helps use glucose from carbohydrates. Cells then use this glucose to produce energy to grow and function. Diabetics are unable to use the sugars they eat because they lack the ability to metabolize them.

Diabetes has been associated with high levels of one particular category of blood fat—the triglycerides. Studies conducted over a ten-year period show that fish-oil supplementation for patients with type II diabetes lowers triglycerides without adversely affecting blood-sugar levels. These data suggest that a marine oil, such as the lipid oil extract of green-lipped mussels, may be safe to add to triglyceride-lowering medication for people with diabetes.

MULTIPLE SCLEROSIS (MS)

The lipid oil extract of green-lipped mussels might be helpful in treating multiple sclerosis (MS), an autoimmune disease that affects the central nervous system (brain and spinal cord). MS occurs when inflammation destroys the insulating myelin sheath that covers the nerve fibers. The nerves lose much of their protective coating. It would be as if the thick plastic coating on phone or electrical wires is stripped away, leaving exposed areas. In the brain, these areas of scarring are called scleroses. The damage in these scleroses slows or blocks muscle coordination, visual sensation, and other nerve signals.

Dr. Sheila Gibson, at the Western Glasgow Hospital in Scotland, has been studying whether green-lipped mussel lipid oil has a beneficial impact on patients with MS who did not respond to any previous treatments. While the effectiveness of the lipid oil extract in combating inflammatory symptoms of MS appears to be logical, only empirical and scientifically valid evidence will prove whether that contention is correct.

DELAYED ONSET MUSCLE SORENESS

Delayed onset muscle soreness (DOMS) is a type-1 muscle strain, with tenderness and stiffness to palpitation and movement one to two days after exercise. It results in a loss of muscle force. For athletes required to train and compete in close succession, DOMS can pose an obstacle to optimal performance. Researchers at the Australian Institute of Sport have enrolled 24 male athletes training at a sub-elite level. They have been subjected to downhill running on a treadmill at 80% of their maximum heart rate and other variables. VAS and readings on an algometer will be performed. Blood samples collected prior to, during, and after exercise will allow for measuring muscular enzymes (CK), acute phase response markers (IL-1, IL-6, IL-10, TNF-alpha, CRP, SAA), skeletal troponins, and white blood cells. The study is a double-blind, placebo-controlled one. The hypothesis is that green-lipped mussel oil will help reduce, or prevent, all abnormal results.

I hope that this chapter has whetted your interest in following news reports emanating from the scientific community regarding the many fascinating applications of the lipid oil of green-lipped mussels. I believe we are living in exciting times and that the studies currently underway are at the cutting edge of modern research into non-pharmaceutical management of chronic illness.

8

How to Use Lipid Oil Extract

We have seen how the lipid oil extract of green-lipped mussels works and what it can do. Now it's time for some practical advice regarding its use.

RECOMMENDED USAGE

Whether you're suffering from arthritis, asthma, or circulatory problems, here's the recommended course of green-lipped mussel lipid oil treatment:

- Clinical trials have shown that the starting dose of 4 capsules a day is recommended as the initial optimum dosage. For consumers with a larger body mass, more severe conditions, or who want quicker results, a higher dose of 4 to 8 capsules should be taken for the initial month.

- After four to six weeks, or after experiencing symptom relief, you can reduce the dosage to 2 or 3 capsules per day or to a level based on personal needs. After another month, you can reduce the dosage even further if warranted.

- A maintenance dose may vary between 1 to 3 capsules a day depending on your body weight/mass and condition.

Among the variables that affect the response to the lipid oil extract is the amount of omega-6 oils you have consumed in the past and that you continue to consume. Also, you need to factor in the number of inflammatory processes at work in your body—allergies, asthma, heart and circulatory problems, diabetes, arthritis, etc.

It takes a month or more for the omega-3 fatty acids in the lipid oil to build up in the body. You must, therefore, take the largest quantity at the beginning of treatment, and then gradually decrease the daily dosage until you have reached a level that maintains the desired effects. The following tips are also helpful when taking this lipid oil:

- You can take the daily dosage with a meal all at once or divide it between morning and evening meals.

- Take lipid oil extract with meals. Some people have reported experiencing mild nausea or belching after taking the oil on an empty stomach.

- Always store lipid oil extract in a cool, dark, dry place.

CAN LIPID OIL EXTRACT OF GREEN-LIPPED MUSSELS BECOME STALE?

The shelf life of most gelatin capsules is usually five years. Theoretically, they are totally weatherproof and impermeable to air. Currently, the oldest batches of lipid oil capsules are six years old, and there has been no degradation and no modification in the capsules. So, we know that after six years the oils are still active, have not been oxidized, and there are no changes.

To be safe, although this lipid oil extract is an antioxidant, the pharmaceutical industry always adds a quarter of a milligram of additional antioxidant (alpha-tocopherol or vitamin E) to soft gelatin capsules. This trace of vitamin E is enough to prevent oxidation. However, the amount of vitamin E in each capsule is minuscule, so do not substitute this vitamin E for your regular vitamin E supplement.

Conclusion

By picking this book up and reading it, you have shown an interest in improving your health, or in helping someone you know who suffers from a chronic inflammatory illness. I hope the information within will, indeed, be helpful to you.

Chronic inflammatory illness is a growing burden. It ruins lives, destroys families, and drains badly needed resources. It may be the price you have to pay for being alive, but no matter how old you are, you should be able to move about freely, hike, garden, swim, or even run whenever you want; you should be able to breathe normally; your body should feel (and be) in shape.

Controlling chronic inflammation is not easy, and requires a strategy. The oil of the green-lipped mussels of New Zealand may well be the major factor to help you enjoy life—and smell the roses. When compared to NSAIDs, aspirin, corticosteroids, beta-agonists, or other prescription drugs, the oil of New Zealand green-lipped mussels, which is available as a supplement, has a flawless safety record. And it is effective, not merely a "Band-Aid" that masks symptoms. Furthermore, it's easy to take: four capsules daily for four to eight weeks, and then one or two capsules a day.

Even if you are not currently suffering from one of the illnesses discussed in this book, I hope that you will consider using this lipid oil preventively. It can only enhance your health. In fact, as the studies have indicated, there really is no "downside" to lipid oil—you cannot overdose on it, nor will it interact negatively with herbs, medications, or other supplements. However, before taking any supplement, you should always discuss it with your health care provider.

As mentioned earlier, the lipid oil extract of green-lipped mussels is not a magic bullet. It works best when incorporated into a broad health-improvement plan, which includes a well-balanced diet, regular exercise, and a low-stress lifestyle. I believe that these recommendations comprise the formula for good health.

In the words of the Maori, *"Kia pai o koutou oranga!"* or "Be in good health!"

Glossary

Acute. Rapid in onset; severe, life-threatening. The opposite of persistent, chronic, or long-term.

Arthritis. Joint inflammation, a group of more than 100 rheumatic diseases that can cause pain, stiffness, and swelling in the joints. These diseases also affect other parts of the body, including muscles, bones, tendons, and ligaments, and some internal organs. The two most common forms of arthritis are osteoarthritis (OA) and rheumatoid arthritis (RA).

Asthma. A chronic inflammatory disorder of the airways in which many cells and cellular elements play a role—in particular, mast cells, eosinophils, T lymphocytes, neutrophils, and epithelial cells.

Allergy. An immediate or delayed immune reaction caused by an allergen—a substance such as dust, a drug, or other foreign material that causes an allergic reaction.

Analgesic. Agent that reduces pain without reducing consciousness.

Antagonist. A drug that prevents or reverses the action of another drug.

Anti-inflammatory. A substance that counteracts or suppresses inflammation. Swelling and redness are signs of inflammation. There are two major types of anti-inflammatory drugs: steroids, such as cortisone, and non-steroidal agents, such as aspirin.

Antioxidant. A substance that neutralizes free radicals that damage the cells and tissues of the body.

Arachidonic acid. An essential fatty acid that is a constituent of human cell membranes. It is also a precursor of some pro-inflammatory body chemicals.

Autoimmune disease. A disease that arises from and is directed against an individual's own tissues.

Cardiovascular system. The heart and blood vessels.

Central nervous system. The main part of the nervous system; includes the brain and spinal cord.

Chronic. Continuous or ongoing.

Diabetes. A condition in which the pancreas produces too little or no insulin, the hormone that enables the cells to absorb glucose. The body becomes unable to use glucose, resulting in major diverse damages, mostly in blood vessels and sensory organs.

Double blind. A type of drug trial in which people are divided into different groups. One group takes the experimental drug and other groups take different doses, the standard therapy, or placebo. Neither the researchers nor the people in the trial know who is taking what until the trial is over.

Drug. According to the definition of the American Medical Association, "a chemical substance that alters the function of one or more body organs or changes the process of a disease." Drugs include prescribed medicines, over-the-counter remedies, and illicit drugs such as cocaine.

Immunoglobulin E (IgE). A class of antibody that is associated with allergy.

Leukotrienes. Chemicals produced within the body that are responsible for initiating and extending the inflammatory process throughout the body. They develop through the lipoxygenase (LOX) pathway.

Lipid. Any of a group of fatty substances including triglycerides (the main forms of fat in body fat), phospholipids (vital constituents of cell membranes), and sterols such as cholesterol.

Placebo. A chemically inactive substance given instead of a drug. In clinical trials, placebos result in clinical improvement in up to 60% of patients.

Prostaglandin. Any of a group of naturally occurring body chemicals, derived from fatty acids, that have a variety of effects, including contraction, inflammation, and damage to tissues.

Symptom. A sign that the body is going through a process. A fever can be a symptom of a more deep-rooted cause—namely, an infection. A rash may be a symptom of an allergy.

Non-steroidal Anti-Inflammatory Drugs (NSAIDs)

The conventional medical treatments for arthritis have largely involved analgesics and non-steroidal anti-inflammatory drugs (NSAIDs). These are designed to control the symptoms of arthritis, including pain and stiffness. Some of these compounds are prescription drugs while others are over-the-counter remedies. The principal and significant drawback of these drugs is their tendency to ulcerate the mucous membranes of the stomach and intestinal tract. Approximately 25% of patients experience one or more of numerous serious side effects, including bleeding ulcers, stomach and intestinal discomfort, liver and kidney problems, and even death.

NSAIDS ON THE MARKET (Prescription and Over-the-Counter)

Aches-N-pain	Anaprox-Ds	Apsifen
Advil	Ansaid	Apsifen-F
Advil Caplets	Apo-Diclo	Bayer Select Pain Relief
Albert-Tiafen	Apo-Flurbiprofen	Formula Caplets
Alka Butazolidin	Apo-Ibuprofen	Brufen
Alkabutazone	Apo-Indomethacin	Butacote
Alka-Phenylbutazone	Apo-Keto	Butazone
Alrheumat	Apo-Keto-E	Children's Advil
Amersol	Apo-Naproxen	Clinoril
Anaprox	Apo-Piroxicam	CoAdvil

Cotybutazone	Indocin SR	Nuprin
Cramp End	Indolar SR	Orudis
Diclofenac	Indomethacin	Orudis-E
Diflunisal	Intrabutazone	Oruvail
Dolgesic	Ketoprofen	Pamprin-IB
Dolobid	Lidifen	Paxofen
Etodolac	Lodine	Pedia
Excedrin-IB	Meclofen	Phenylbutazone
Feldene	Meclofenamate	Phenylone Plus
Fenoprofen	Meclomen	Piroxicam
Fenopron	Medipren	Ponstan
Flurbiprofen	Mefenamic Acid	Ponstel
Froben	Midol 200	Progesic
Genpril	Midol IB	Relafen
Haltran	Motrin	Rhodis-EC
Ibifon 600	Motrin IB	Rufen
Ibren	Motrin IB caplets	Saleto-200
Ibu	Motrin, Children's	Saleto-400
Ibu-4	Nabumetone	Saleto-600
Ibu-6	Nalfon	Saleto-800
Ibu-8	Nalfon 200	Sulindac
Ibu-200	Naprosyn	Surgam
Ibumed	Naproxen	Synflex
Ibuprin	Naxen	Telectin DS
Ibupro-600	Novobutazone	Tenoxicam
Ibuprofen	Novo-Keto-EC	Tiaprofenic acid
Ibutex	Novomethacin	Tolmetin
Ifen	Novonaprox	Trendar
Imbrilon	Novopirocam	Voltaren
Indameth	Novoprofen	Voltaren SR
Indocid	Novo-Sundac	Voltarol
Indocid SR	Nu-Indo	Voltarol Retard
Indocin	Nu-Pirox	

Selected References

Adler, A.J., and B.J. Holub. "Effect of Garlic and Fish-Oil Supplementation on Serum Lipid and Lipoprotein Concentrations in Hypercholesterolemic Men." *American Journal of Clinical Nutrition* 64(1997): 445–450.

Antileukotriene Working Group, et al. *Asthma 2000—The Role of Antileukotrienes in Clinical Practice.* Discovery International, 1999.

Audeval, B., and P. Bouchacourt. "Etude controlée, en double aveugle contre placebo, de l'extrait de moule *Perna canaliculus* (moule aux orles verts) dans la gonarthrose." *La Gazette Médicale* 93.

Bang, H.O., and J. Dyerberg. "Plasma Lipids and Lipoproteins in Greenlandic West Coast Eskimos." *Acta Medica Scandinavica* 192(1972): 85–94.

Belluzzi, A., S. Boschi, C. Brignola, et al. "Polyunsaturated Fatty Acids and Inflammatory Bowel Disease." *American Journal of Clinical Nutrition* 71(2000):339S–342S.

Bhathena, S.J., E. Berlin, J. T. Judd, et al. "Effects of Omega-3 Fatty Acids and Vitamin E on Hormones Involved in Carbohydrate and Lipid Metabolism in Men." *American Journal of Clinical Nutrition* 54 (1991):684–688.

Blonk, M.C., H.J. Bilo, J.J. Nauta, et al. "Dose-Response Effects of Fish-Oil Supplementation in Healthy Volunteers." *American Journal of Clinical Nutrition* 52(1990):120–127.

Burr, M.L. "Lessons from the Story of Omega-3 Fatty Acids." *American Journal of Clinical Nutrition* 71(2000):397S–398S.

Cho, S.H., Y.B. Jung, S.C. Seong, et al. "Clinical Efficacy and Safety of Lyprinol, a Patented Extract from New Zealand Green-lipped Mussel (*Perna canaliculus*) in Patients with Osteoarthritis of the Hip and Knee: A Multicenter 2-month Clinical Trial." *Allergie & Immunologie* (Paris) 35(2003):212–216.

Cobiac, L., P.M. Clifton, M. Abbey, et al. "Lipid, Lipoprotein, and Hemostatic Effects of Fish vs. Fish-Oil Omega-3 Fatty Acids in Mildly Hyperlipidemic Males." *American Journal of Clinical Nutrition* 53(1991): 1210–1216.

Connor, S.L., and W.E. Connor. "Are Fish Oils Beneficial in the Prevention and Treatment of Coronary Artery Disease?" *American Journal of Clinical Nutrition* 66(1997):1020S–1031S.

Connor, W. E. "Importance of Omega-3 Fatty Acids in Health and Disease." *American Journal of Clinical Nutrition* 71(2000):171S–175S.

Connor, W.E., and A. Bendich, eds. "Highly Unsaturated Fatty Acids in Nutrition and Disease Prevention." Proceedings of a Conference Held in Barcelona, Spain (November 4–6, 1996). Supplement to *American Journal of Clinical Nutrition* 71(2000).

Dannenberg, A.J., and D. Zakim. "Chemoprevention of Colorectal Cancer Through Inhibition of Cyclooxygenase-2." *Seminars in Oncology* 26 (1999):499–504.

Donadio, J.V., Jr. "Use of Fish Oil to Treat Patients with Immunoglobulin A Nephropathy." *American Journal of Clinical Nutrition* 71(2000): 373S–375S.

Dugas, B. "Lyprinol Inhibits LTB$_4$ Production by Human Monocytes." *Allergie & Immunologie* 32(2000):284–289.

Emelyanov, A., G. Fedoseev, O. Krasnoschekova, et al. "Treatment of Asthma with Lipid Extract of New Zealand Green-lipped Mussel: A Randomised Clinical Trial." *European Respiratory Journal* 20(2002): 596–600.

Fernandez, E., L. Chatenoud, C. La Vecchia, et al. "Fish Consumption and Cancer Risk." *American Journal of Clinical Nutrition* 70(1999):85–90.

Flaten, H., A.T. Hostmark, P. Kierulf, et al. "Fish-Oil Concentrate: Effects on Variables Related to Cardiovascular Disease." *American Journal of Clinical Nutrition* 52(1990):300–306.

Gibson, R.G., S.L.M.Gibson, V. Conway, et al. "*Perna canaliculus* in the Treatment of Arthritis." *The Practitioner* 224(1980):955–960.

Gibson, S.L.M., and R.G. Gibson. "The Treatment of Arthritis with a Lipid Extract of *Perna canaliculus:* A Randomized Trial." *Complementary Therapies in Medicine* 6(1998):122.

Gruenwald, J., H. J. Graubaum, K. Hansen, et al. "Efficacy and Tolerability of a Combination of Lyprinol and High Concentrations of EPA and DHA in Inflammatory Rheumatoid Disorders." *Advances in Therapy* 21(2004):197–201.

Halpern, G.M. "Anti-inflammatory Effects of a Stabilized Lipid Extract of *Perna canaliculus* (Lyprinol)." *Allergie & Immunologie* 32(2000):272–278.

Halpern, G.M. "Recent Advances in Human Nutrition and the Science of Pleasure." Published in part in *EAACI Newsletter* 2–3(1999):4–7.

Halpern, G.M. *Ulcer Free!* Garden City Park, NY: Square One Publishers, 2004.

Harris, W.S. "Omega-3 Fatty Acids and Serum Lipoproteins: Animal Studies." *American Journal of Clinical Nutrition* 65(1997):1611S–1616S.

Harris, W.S. "Omega-3 Fatty Acids and Serum Lipoproteins: Human Studies." *American Journal of Clinical Nutrition* 65(1997):1645S–1654S.

Herold, P.M., and J.E. Kinsella. "Fish Oil Consumption and Decreased Risk of Cardiovascular Disease: A Comparison of Findings from Animal and Human Feeding Trials." *American Journal of Clinical Nutrition* 43(1986):566–598.

Holgate, S.X, and M.K.Church. *Allergy.* London and New York: Gower Medical Publishing, 1993.

Hooper, S. "The Effect of Marine Oils on Markers of Thrombosis in the Blood of Healthy Females." Bachelor of Applied Science (Honours) Thesis, Department of Medical Laboratory Science (Haematology), Faculty of Biomedical and Health Sciences and Nursing, RMIT University, Australia (October 1998).

Hwang, D.H., P.S. Chanmugam, D.H. Ryan, et al. "Does Vegetable Oil Attenuate the Beneficial Effects of Fish Oil in Reducing Risk Factors for Cardiovascular Disease?" *American Journal of Clinical Nutrition* 66(1997):89–96.

James, M.L., R.A. Gibson, and L.G. Cleland. "Dietary Polyunsaturated Fatty Acids and Inflammatory Mediator Production." *American Journal of Clinical Nutrition* 71(2000):343S–348S.

Katan, M.B., P.L. Zock, and R.P. Mensink. "Effects of Fats and Fatty Acids on Blood Lipids in Humans: An Overview." *American Journal of Clinical Nutrition* 60(1994):1017S–1022S.

Kremer, J.M. "Omega-3 Fatty Acid Supplements in Rheumatoid Arthritis." *American Journal of Clinical Nutrition* 71(2000):349S–351S.

Lau, C.S., P.K.Y. Chiu, E.M.Y. Chu, et al. "Treatment of Knee Osteoarthritis with Lyprinol, Lipid Extract of the Green-lipped Mussel—A Double-blind Placebo-controlled Study." *Progress in Nutrition* 6(2004): 17–31.

Ludwig, D.S., K.E. Peterson, and S.L. Gortmaker. "Relation Between Consumption of Sugar-Sweetened Drinks and Childhood Obesity: A Prospective, Observational Analysis." *Lancet* 357(2001):505–508.

Mathews-Roth, M.M. "Carotenoids in Erythropoietic Protoporphyria and Other Photosensitivity Diseases." *Annals of the New York Academy of Sciences* 691(1993):127–138.

Murphy K.J., K. Galvin, M. Kiely, et al. "Can Dietary Supplementation with the New Zealand Green-lipped Mussel (NZGLM) Reduce Pro-inflammatory Eicosanoids and Cytokines in vivo?" Accepted for publication in *European Journal of Clinical Nutrition.*

Murphy, K.J., B.D. Mooney, N.J. Mann, et al. "Lipid, FA, and Sterol Composition of New Zealand Green-lipped Mussel (*Perna canaliculus*) and Tasmanian Blue Mussel (*Mytilus edulis*)." *Lipids* 37(2002):587–595.

Naikhin, A.N., A.R. Rekstin, S.A. Donina, et al. "Immune Response to Live Influenza Vaccine." *Vestn Ross Akad Med Nauk* (in Russian) 12(2002):24–28.

Natarajan, R., and J. Nadler. "Role of Lipoxygenase in Breast Cancer." *Frontiers in Bioscience* 3(1998):E81–E88.

National Institutes of Health. "Global Initiative for Asthma—Global Strategy for Asthma Management and Prevention NHLBI/WHO Workshop Report, March 1995," Publication No. 95-3659. Washington, DC: National Institutes of Health, 1995.

Nestel, P.J. "Fish Oil and Cardiovascular Disease: Lipids and Arterial Function." *American Journal of Clinical Nutrition* 71(2000):228–231.

Rainsford, K.D., and M.W. Whitehouse. "Gastroprotective and Anti-inflammatory Properties of Green-Lipped Mussel (*Perna canaliculus*) Preparation." *Arzneimittelforschung* 30(1980):2128–2132.

Shiels, I.A., and M.W. Whitehouse. "Lyprinol: Anti-inflammatory and Uterine Relaxant Activities in Rats, with Special Reference to a Model for Dysmenorrhea." *Allergie & Immunologie* 32(2000):279–283.

Sinclair, A.J., K.J. Murphy, and D. Li. "Marine Lipids: Overview: New Insights, and Lipid Composition of Lyprinol." *Allergie & Immunologie* 32(2000):261–271.

Speed, A., and D. Zwar. "Introducing: The Ocean Mussel That Packs a Punch Against Arthritis Pain." *Bio/Tech News* (1997).

Tenikoff, D., K.J. Murphy, M. Le, et al. "Lyprinol: A Potential Preventive Treatment for Inflammatory Bowel Disease (IBD)." *Pacific Journal of Clinical Nutrition* 13 Suppl(2004):S94.

Turcios, N. L. "What You Need to Know about Pediatric Asthma Pharmacology." *Contemporary Pediatrics* 8(2002):101.

Whitehouse, M.W. "Adjuvant-Induced Polyarthritis in Rats." In *CRC Handbook of Animal Models for the Rheumatic Diseases* Vol. 1, edited by R. A. Greenwald and H. S. Diamond. Miami, FL: CRC Press, 1996.

Whitehouse, M.W. "Non-NSAID Over-the-Counter Remedies for Arthritis: Which Are the Good, the Bad, the Indifferent?" SEADS/Inflammopharmacology Meeting, Georgia, May 1999.

Whitehouse, M.W., T.A. Macrides, N. Kalafatis, et al. "Anti-inflammatory Activity of a Lipid Fraction (Lyprinol) from the N. Z. Green-Lipped Mussel." *Inflammopharmacology* 5(1997):237–246.

Whitehouse, M.W., M.S. Roberts, and P.M. Brooks. "Over-the-Counter (OTC) Oral Remedies for Arthritis and Rheumatism: How Effective Are They?" *Inflammopharmacology* 7(1999):89–105.

Whitehouse, M.W. "Anti-TNF-alpha Therapy for Chronic Inflammation: Reconsidering Pentoxiphylline as an Alternative to Therapeutic Protein Drugs." *Inflammopharmacology* 12(2004):223–227.

About the Author

Georges M. Halpern, MD, PhD, is Distinguished Professor of Pharmaceutical Sciences at the Hong Kong Polytechnic University, Honorary Professor of Pharmacology at the University of Hong Kong, and past Professor of Medicine at the University of California, at Davis.

Dr. Halpern was born a French citizen in Warsaw, Poland, and attended medical school at the University of Paris. In 1964, he received his MD degree and was awarded a silver medal for his thesis. He subsequently qualified in nuclear medicine and was board certified in internal medicine and allergy. In 1992, he received his PhD degree, with highest honors and jury honors, from the Faculty of Pharmacy at the University of Paris XI. He was recently promoted to the rank of Commander in the French National Order of the Mérite Agricole for his original contributions to French cuisine and enology.

Dr. Halpern has published seventeen books, many book chapters, original papers, and hundreds of reviews and abstracts. He has lectured in seventy-six countries. In 1985, he was awarded the Medal of Vermeil by the city of Paris for his outstanding contributions to medicine, dedication to patients, and personal achievements.

Dr. Halpern is a Fellow of the American Academy of Allergy, Asthma, and Immunology and a member of twenty-six other academies and scientific societies. He resides in Portola Valley, California.

Index

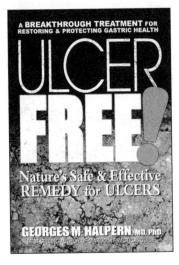

ULCER FREE!
Nature's Safe and Effective Remedy for Ulcers
Georges M. Halpern, MD

Over 4 million Americans are diagnosed annually with peptic ulcer disease. Many learn to live with the resulting heartburn, acid reflux, nausea, gas, and stomach pain with the help of over-the-counter antacids. These products may stop the pain, but only temporarily. Furthermore, the underlying condition can worsen. But it doesn't have to be that way. *Ulcer Free!* is a practical guide to understanding the causes of and effective treatments for peptic ulcer disease.

The book begins with a look at why we get ulcers. It examines the *Helicobacter pylori* bacterium—the culprit behind the majority of stomach ulcers. It also discusses the growing number of ulcers caused by NSAIDs—over-the-counter pain relievers, more commonly known as aspirin, ibuprofen, naproxen, and a variety of other products. The book then offers an unbiased look at the treatments—conventional and alternative—that can stop the symptoms of and actually heal ulcers. Finally, *Ulcer Free!* introduces the breakthrough nutrient Zinc-Carnosine, which can be used in conjunction with other treatments or on its own.

If you are tired of being victim to continual gastric distress, *Ulcer Free!* can help. Up-to-date and accurate, it offers the key to permanent relief.

Georges M. Halpern, MD, attended medical school at the University of Paris, France. He subsequently received a PhD from the Faculty of Pharmacy, University of Paris XI—Chatenay Malabry. A Fellow of the American Academy of Allergy and Immunology, Dr. Halpern is board certified in internal medicine and allergy, and is Professor Emeritus of Medicine at the University of California—Davis. He is also a Distinguished Professor of Medicine at the University of Hong Kong.

$14.95 • 208 pages • 6 x 9-inch quality paperback • ISBN 0-7570-0253-6

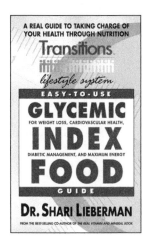

GLYCEMIC INDEX FOOD GUIDE

For Weight Loss, Cardiovascular Health, Diabetic Management, and Maximum Energy

Dr. Shari Lieberman

The glycemic index (GI) is an important nutritional tool. By indicating how quickly a given food triggers a rise in blood sugar, the GI enables you to choose foods that can help you manage a variety of conditions, as well as improve your overall health.

Whether you are interested in controlling your glucose levels to manage your diabetes, lose weight, increase your heart health, boost your energy level, or simply enhance your well-being, *Transitions Lifestyle System Glycemic Index Food Guide* is the best place to start.

$7.95 U.S. • 160 pages • 4 x 7-inch mass paperback • ISBN 978-0-7570-0245-8

THE ACID ALKALINE FOOD GUIDE

A Quick Reference to Foods & Their Effect on pH Levels

Dr. Susan E. Brown and Larry Trivieri, Jr.

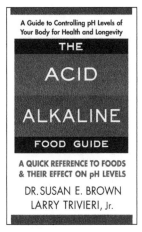

In the last few years, researchers around the world have reported the importance of acid-alkaline balance to good health. While thousands of people are trying to balance their body's pH level, until now, they have had to rely on guides containing only a small number of foods. *The Acid-Alkaline Food Guide* is a complete resource for people who want to widen their food choices.

The book begins by explaining how the acid-alkaline environment of the body is influenced by foods. It then presents a list of thousands of foods—single foods, combination foods, and even fast foods—and their acid-alkaline effects. *The Acid-Alkaline Food Guide* will quickly become the resource you turn to at home, in restaurants, and whenever you want to select a food that can help you reach your health and dietary goals.

$7.95 U.S. • 208 pages • 4 x 7-inch mass paperback • ISBN 978-0-7570-0280-9

THE MAGNESIUM SOLUTION FOR HIGH BLOOD PRESSURE
How to Use Magnesium to Help Prevent and Relieve Hypertension Naturally

Jay S. Cohen, MD

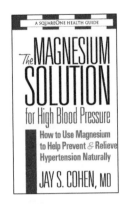

Approximately 50 percent of all Americans have hypertension, a devastating disease that can lead to hardening of the arteries, heart attack, and stroke. While many medications are available to combat this condition, these drugs come with potentially dangerous side effects. When Dr. Jay S. Cohen learned of his own hypertension, he was well aware of the risks associated with standard treatments. Based upon his research, he selected a safer option—magnesium.

In *The Magnesium Solution for High Blood Pressure,* Dr. Cohen describes the most effective types of magnesium for treating hypertension, explores appropriate magnesium dosage, and details the use of magnesium in conjunction with hypertension meds. Here is a proven remedy for anyone looking for a safe, effective approach to the treatment of high blood pressure.

$5.95 • 96 pages • 4 x 7-inch mass paperback • ISBN 0-7570-0255-2

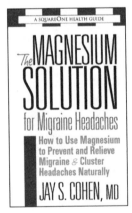

THE MAGNESIUM SOLUTION FOR MIGRAINE HEADACHES
How to Use Magnesium to Prevent and Relieve Migraine and Cluster Headaches Naturally

Jay S. Cohen, MD

More than 30 million people across North America suffer from migraine headaches. Over the years, a number of drugs have been developed to treat migraines, but these treatments don't work for everyone, and come with a high risk of side effects. Fortunately, Dr. Jay S. Cohen has discovered an alternative—magnesium.

This easy-to-understand guide explains what a migraine is, and shows how this supplement can play a key role in preventing and treating migraine headaches. It also describes what type of magnesium works best, and how much magnesium should be taken to prevent or stop migraines. For those who are looking for a safe and effective approach to the prevention and treatment of migraine and cluster headaches, Dr. Cohen prescribes a proven natural remedy in *The Magnesium Solution for Migraine Headaches.*

$5.95 • 96 pages • 4 x 7-inch mass paperback • ISBN 0-7570-0256-0

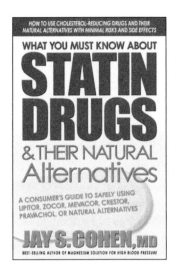

WHAT YOU MUST KNOW ABOUT STATIN DRUGS & THEIR NATURAL ALTERNATIVES

A Consumer's Guide to Safely Using Lipitor, Zocor, Mevacor, Crestor, Pravachol, or Natural Alternatives

Jay S. Cohen, MD

It is estimated that over 100 million Americans suffer from elevated cholesterol and C-reactive proteins—markers that are linked to heart attack, stroke, and other cardiovascular disorders. To combat these problems, modern science has created a group of drugs known either as statins or as specific commercial drugs such as Lipitor, Zocor, and Pravachol. While over 20 million people take these medications, the fact is that up to 42 percent experience side effects, and a whopping 60 to 70 percent eventually stop treatment. Here, for the first time, is a guide that explains the problems caused by statins, and offers easy-to-follow strategies that will allow you to benefit from these drugs while avoiding their side effects. In addition, the author provides natural alternatives that have also proven effective.

What You Must Know About Statin Drugs & Their Natural Alternatives begins by explaining elevated cholesterol and C-reactive proteins. It then examines how statins work to alleviate these problems, and discusses possible side effects. Highlighted is information on safe usage, as well as a discussion of effective alternative treatments. If you have elevated cholesterol and C-reactive proteins, or if you are currently using a statin, *What You Must Know About Statin Drugs & Their Natural Alternatives* can make a profound difference in the quality of your life.

Jay S. Cohen, MD, is an Associate Professor (voluntary) of Family and Preventive Medicine and of Psychiatry at the University of California, San Diego, where he teaches medical students and staff. For over thirteen years, Dr. Cohen has specialized in psychopharmacology. Since 1990, he has conducted research on drugs and their side effects. He is the author of numerous research papers, published articles, and books, including *Over Dose: The Case Against the Drug Companies.* Dr. Cohen currently lives in Del Mar, California.

$15.95 • 224 pages • 6 x 9-inch paperback • ISBN 0-7570-0257-9

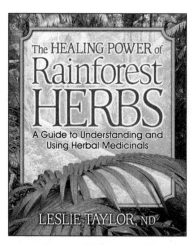

THE HEALING POWER OF RAINFOREST HERBS

A Guide to Understanding and Using Herbal Medicinals

Leslie Taylor, ND

Rainforests contain an amazing abundance of plant life—just two-and-a-half acres of Amazon rainforest are believed to house approximately 900 tons of botanicals. Even more exciting is the fact that scientists and researchers have only just begun to uncover the medicinal properties of rainforest herbs and flora. Nature has provided us with a treasure of herbal remedies—secrets that offer new approaches to health and healing. *The Healing Power of Rainforest Herbs* is a valuable guide to these herbs and their uses.

Detailing more than fifty rainforest botanicals, *The Healing Power of Rainforest Herbs* is the result of years of extensive research by naturopath Leslie Taylor. In it, she explains the medicinal properties of each herb and the natural chemicals involved, as well as preparation instructions. The author has also included the history of the herbs' use by indigenous peoples, and their current usage by natural health practitioners around the world. Helpful tables provide a quick guide to choosing the most useful botanicals for specific ailments. Illustrations of plants and recipes for herbal remedies complete the wealth of information found in this resource.

The Healing Power of Rainforest Herbs offers a blend of ancient and modern knowledge in an accessible reference guide. This unique book incorporates the healing practices of shamans with scientific research for anyone seeking to discover the medicinal secrets of the rainforest.

Leslie Taylor, ND, survived a rare form of leukemia by following alternative and herbal medicinal therapies. A practicing herbalist and naturopath, Dr. Taylor has been researching, studying, and documenting herbal medicine for almost twenty years. She is the founder of Raintree Nutrition Inc., a company dedicated to making rainforest botanicals available while preserving the rainforests from destruction. Dr. Taylor lectures and teaches classes worldwide in naturopathic medicine, herbal medicine, ethnobotany, and environmental and sustainability issues.

$18.95 • 268 pages • 7.5 x 9-inch quality paperback • ISBN 0-7570-0144-0

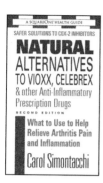

Natural Alternatives to Vioxx, Celebrex

& Other Anti-Inflammatory Prescription Drugs

Carol Simontacchi

Beyond today's headlines is an underlying truth—COX-2 inhibitors can be dangerous to your health. This guide points the way to far safer alternatives. It first examines the cause of arthritis pain, and then discusses the most effective supplements available for the treatment of this condition. Here is a vital resource for those looking for a better solution.

$5.95 • 128 pages • 4 x 7-inch mass paperback • ISBN 978-0-7570-0278-6

Natural Alternatives to Lipitor, Zocor & Other Statin Drugs

Jay S. Cohen, MD

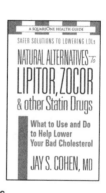

Elevated cholesterol and C-reactive proteins are markers linked to heart attack, stroke, and other cardiovascular disorders. While modern science has created a group of drugs known as statins to combat these problems, nearly 50 percent of the people who take them experience side effects. This guide explains the problems caused by statins and highlights the most effective natural alternatives.

$7.95 • 144 pages • 4 x 7-inch mass paperback • ISBN 978-0-7570-0286-1

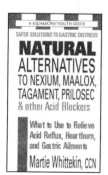

Natural Alternatives to Nexium, Maalox, Tagament, Prilosec

& Other Acid Blockers

Martie Whittekin, CCN

Natural Alternatives to Nexium, Maalox, Tagament, Prilosec & Other Acid Blockers begins by examining how acid blockers work, and discusses possible long-range side effects. It then explains those underlying causes of the problem that can be corrected. Finally, the author highlights the most important natural alternatives. If you suffer from the pain of recurrent gastric upset, or if you are currently using an acid blocker, *Natural Alternatives* can make a profound difference in the quality of your life.

$7.95 • 160 pages • 4 x 7-inch mass paperback • ISBN 978-0-7570-0210-6

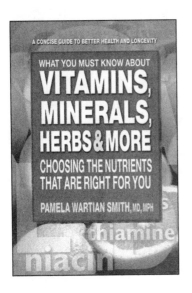

WHAT YOU MUST KNOW ABOUT VITAMINS, MINERALS, HERBS & MORE

Choosing the Nutrients
That Are Right for You

Pamela Wartian Smith, MD, MPH

Almost 75 percent of your health and life expectancy is based on lifestyle, environment, and nutrition. Yet even if you follow a healthful diet, you are probably not getting all the nutrients you need to prevent disease. In *What You Must Know About Vitamins, Minerals, Herbs & More,* Dr. Pamela Smith explains how you can restore and maintain health through the wise use of nutrients.

Part One of this easy-to-use guide discusses the individual nutrients necessary for good health. Part Two offers personalized nutritional programs for people with a wide variety of health concerns. People without prior medical problems can look to Part Three for their supplementation plans. Whether you want to maintain good health or you are trying to overcome a medical condition, *What You Must Know About Vitamins, Minerals, Herbs & More* can help you make the best choices for the health and well-being of you and your family.

$15.95 • 448 pages • 6 x 9-inch quality paperback • ISBN 978-0-7570-0233-5